The Miracle of **MSM**

g. p. putnam's sons · new york

To my beloved children—Stephen, Jeffrey, Darren, Robert, and Elyse.

—Stanley Jacob, M.D.

To Eleanor, Michele, Lesli, Stewart, Allison, and Jeremy.

—Ronald M. Lawrence, M.D., Ph.D.

To Rosita, my precious soul mate, for patience, support, and love.

—Martin Zucker

Acknowledgments

The authors would like to express gratitude to the many people who helped in the making of this book:

To Jack Scovil, literary agent extraordinaire, for foresight, insight, guidance and good humor.

To Stacy Creamer, our editor, for keeping us firmly focused and making many winning suggestions.

To the following individuals who generously shared with the authors their personal experiences for the purpose of giving hope to others in pain: Sue Ellen Andrus; Helen Brant; Joe Bryan; Cheryl Brown; Dick Brown; Father Sam Bungo; Charlotte Callan; Lynne Chauncey; James Coburn; Carol Davis; Linda Dickter; Dan Drown; Katherine Dubik; Mary and Albert Duell; Chris Dugan; Joe Durkee; Helle Ebbesen; James Fitzsimmons, M.D.; Maggie Fredericks; Haruo "Foozie" Fujisawa; Marian Gormley-Pekkola; Cindy Honaker; Ruth Ann Hubler; Margaret Itow; Stephen Jacob; Joyce Jensen; June Jones; Kaye Kolkmann; Gail Lind; Richard Liss; Paul Lisseck; Scott Magers; Pekka Mero; Fritz Meyer; Dorothy Miller; Liz and Ken Miners; Douglas Molnar; Ellen Nelson; Barbara Norman; Doug Ohmart; Alondra Oubre, Ph.D; Nick and Vincenza Puccio; Barbara Redmond; Thomas

Reilly; Bill Rich; Jeff Roake; Michele Robinson, L.P.N.; Tom Rodriquez; Angela Driscoll Ryan, R.N.; Lou Salyer; Laura Scozzaro, L.P.N.; Linda Scotson; Joyce Scott; Gary Sebring; Melvin Shiota; Frank Smith; Beverly Spencer; Lyn Stadish, M.D.; J. Tomita; Sue Watson; Nic Wickliff; Hermine Zubko.

To the following clinicians for sharing their observations on MSM: David Blyweiss, M.D., of the Institute of Advanced Medicine in Lauderhill, Florida; Stacy Childs, M.D., of Cheyenne, Wyoming; Jeffrey Marrongelle, D.C., Schuylkill Haven, Pennsylvania; Trent Nichols, M.D., of the Center for Nutrition and Digestive Disorders in Hanover, Pennsylvania; Efrain Olszewer, M.D., of the International Preventive Medicine Clinic of São Paulo, Brazil; Richard Schaefer, D.C., Wheeling, Illinois; John L. Tate, D.D.S., Spartanburg, South Carolina; Craig Zunka, D.D.S., Front Royal, Virginia.

To the following individuals for sharing valued expertise: Vivien Gore Allen, Ph.D., professor of plant and soil science at Texas Tech University; Siegward Elsas, M.D., Department of Neurology of the UCLA School of Medicine; Maria C. Linder, professor of biochemistry, California State University at Fullerton; Eric S. Saltzman, Ph.D., professor of marine and atmospheric chemistry, University of Miami; Dana Ullman, M.P.H.; nutritional researchers Melvyn Werbach, M.D., and Jeffrey Moss, D.D.S.

To the following individuals for ideas, inspiration and assistance in locating MSM users: Rex Bailey; Arkie Barlet; Bill Fleet; Cindy Kornspan; John Turner; Joan and Lydia Wilen.

To Rita Randall, Jessica Whorton, Marion Odell, and Gwen Crippen for administrative assistance.

And to Roger Cathey for superb fact-finding, critical reviews, and conceptualizing under pressure.

Note to the Reader

This book about the nutritional supplement MSM is not intended as medical advice and should not be used to replace medical care or any therapeutic program recommended by a physician. It is meant for information and education only.

If you have symptoms or suffer from an illness, you should consult with an appropriate health professional for your condition.

If you are currently taking prescription drugs, do not discontinue them or replace them based on any of the information or recommendations appearing in this book without first consulting your doctor.

Clinical experience indicates that MSM does not interfere with any medication. However, if you are under treatment for any condition and are considering taking MSM, we recommend that you first inform your physician and obtain his or her opinion.

The authors invite correspondence from readers describing personal experiences with MSM. Include an address and phone number with the letter, and mail to: MSM, PO Box 447, Agoura Hills, CA 91376-0447. Readers with questions about MSM are also welcome to write to the same address. Please include a self-addressed stamped envelope that can be used for the reply.

Foreword

You are about to read a report on MSM, a nutritional supplement attracting widespread excitement similar to the enthusiasm I witnessed a few years ago with the publication of my books on melatonin and DHEA.

MSM appears to be another natural substance promising substantial benefits, such as relief from pain, inflammation, and allergies, for those who take it as a nutritional supplement.

As a physician, my concern for patient care always involves the fundamental principle of "Do no harm." Unfortunately, in our efforts to help patients with disability and discomfort, we often rely on medications that have significant toxicity and create adverse side effects.

As a medical oncologist and gerontologist, I am always skeptical of the value of a nontoxic drug, but many vitamins and food supplements have a place in medicine as substances offering therapeutic effects without major clinical toxicity. The use of agents such as melatonin and MSM is giving health professionals new, safer options with which to help combat the debility of chronic disease.

MSM is nontoxic! Preliminary studies and the many testimonials reported in this text from people who have taken MSM, even for chronic, severe, and long-term conditions, give us tantalizing evidence of a form of relief that the medical community should take seriously.

I have known Dr. Stanley Jacob for many years and am familiar with his outstanding work at the Oregon Health Sciences University in Portland, where he has treated thousands of patients with severe pain. I became interested in MSM because of my long-standing knowledge of its parent compound, DMSO, which over the years has clearly demonstrated its value throughout the world for uses as varied as pain relief, head trauma, scleroderma, interstitial cystitis, rheumatoid arthritis and osteoarthritis, retransformation of cancer cells, and Alzheimer's disease.

MSM is an odorless metabolite of DMSO! It is a nontoxic relative of its parent compound. Does it have some of the numerous physiologic effects of DMSO? Time will provide the full answer to this question. I do feel that the combined clinical experiences reported in this book by doctors Jacob and Lawrence, along with the myriad of anecdotal reports they have collected, give a promising picture of significant validity regarding MSM's pain and inflammatory relieving effects. I hope this book will stimulate larger controlled clinical trials. Perhaps the Office of Alternative Medicine at the National Institutes of Health will be inspired to conduct such research that will yield greater understanding of the mechanisms and potential of MSM. Until such studies are completed, we have to depend on the detailed experiences reported in this book.

Each patient is an individual and tends to respond differently to the same drug or supplement. But as you read the vast collection of data and reports in this text, you will learn that MSM appears to be safe and is helping many people.

If you do try MSM, keep your physician informed and follow the thoughtful instructions in the book. Your physician will ask if MSM is a safe and effective nutritional supplement. Read the book! I feel the information presented suggests an answer. How-

ever, only your experience can establish the validity of the claims
for MSM.

                         —William Regelson, M.D.
                           professor of medicine,
                           Virginia Commonwealth University
                           Richmond, Virginia,
                           and co-author of *The Melatonin Miracle*
                           and *The Super-Hormone Promise*

Part ONE

ABC's of MSM

took months, MSM first cleared up most of the pain and then the massive inflammation of her jaw joint, allowing her to resume a normal life.

● A Canadian researcher with chronic tendinitis of the arm, and his wife, a hairdresser who had developed back pain from years of standing and serving customers in her beauty salon, were both relieved of their pain with MSM.

The foregoing cases, covered in greater detail later in the book, are a tip of the iceberg, an indication of the broad pain-relieving potential of MSM.

Clinical experience involving thousands of cases has demonstrated that MSM provides relief in about 70 percent of patients with pain. Given the massive incidence of pain problems in our society, this suggests a huge role for MSM if it were to be recommended by physicians as an addition to their regular treatment of pain. MSM certainly fits the growing demand of patients seeking alternative remedies that do not cause adverse side effects.

The Pain Epidemic

In the U.S., pain has reached "epidemic" proportions, according to a July 1997 *Science News Report* issued by the American Medical Association. Citing Norman J. Marcus, M.D., director of the New York Pain Treatment Program at Lenox Hill Hospital in New York City, the report said that "tens of millions of Americans suffer from some form of pain each year, taking a substantial toll on their productivity in the workplace and their ability to take care of their responsibilities at home."

According to *The Management of Pain,* a two-volume reference book for physicians published in 1990, more than one-third of the American population have chronic painful conditions and of those, half or more are partially or totally disabled for periods of days, weeks, months, years, or permanently.

Such pain comes in many forms:

- Headaches that disrupt productivity among 40 million Americans each year.

- Back pain suffered by 36 million people.

- Arthritis afflicting more than 40 million individuals. This includes degenerative arthritis (osteoarthritis), the most common type, 21 million sufferers; fibromyalgia, affecting 3 to 6 million; and rheumatoid arthritis, the most crippling type of the illness, 2.5 million.

- Neck pain—20 million.

- Another 24 million people are debilitated in some way by muscle pain.

- Other painful disorders—neurologic, cardiac, cancer, facial, and abdominal—involve more than 11 million.

- So-called repetitive strain injuries (RSIs) affect the hands, arms, shoulders, necks and backs of countless workers who constantly repeat the same motions day after day, year after year, motions such as gripping, twisting, bending, lifting, reaching, cutting, and keying. Unlike a sudden accident, these overuse conditions develop slowly and cause minute trauma to muscles, tendons, joints, and nerves. Over time, the damage builds up into severe pain, numbness, inflammation, restriction of joint movement, loss of strength and manual dexterity, arthritic conditions, and, if left untreated, lasting disability. According to the U.S. Bureau of Labor Statistics, RSIs account for about 60 percent—and rank first—among all work-caused physical illnesses.

- The medical cost of disability, as well as loss of productivity, is estimated at more than $100 billion per year for persistent pain.

The Side-Effects Epidemic

Treatment of pain typically revolves around pharmaceutical drugs and has contributed to sales that have made the pharmaceutical industry the nation's most profitable as measured by return on investment. While many conditions are so painfully severe that they require powerful medication, there is a serious downside to widespread usage—the issue of safety. Adverse reactions to medical drugs are believed responsible for more than 100,000 deaths and 1.5 million hospitalizations in the U.S. each year, according to reports in the *Journal of the American Medical Association* and other leading medical publications. Fatal drug reactions are, in fact, among the leading causes of death.

Medical authorities continually caution physicians and patients alike regarding the use of nonsteroidal anti-inflammatories (NSAIDs) for pain conditions. They frequently cause ulcers, serious side effects, and even fatalities. Recently, one such drug was removed from the market shortly after it was approved because of four deaths and illness necessitating liver transplants among eight of its users.

Many of our patients come to us with drug-induced symptoms. They are often unable to continue taking NSAIDs prescribed by other physicians because they cannot tolerate the side effects of stomach pangs, acid reflux, and nausea.

Steroidal drugs such as cortisone are also widely prescribed to reduce the inflammation associated with a wide array of painful conditions. These are important drugs but they frequently lead to unhealthy weight gain, high blood pressure, a characteristic "moon face," and even diabetes.

MSM—Relief Without Side Effects

Two of us (Jacob and Lawrence) are medical doctors with nearly ninety years of combined clinical experience treating severe and debilitating pain problems. One of us (Jacob) participated in the development of MSM and was the first physician to use MSM in the treatment of patients nearly twenty years ago. We have both repeatedly seen MSM significantly ease the suffering of patients with different types of pain and inflammatory conditions and restore their ability to function more normally. In our opinion, MSM can greatly reduce the staggering amount of disability and loss of productivity caused by chronic pain.

People continually tell us:

- "I wish I had had known about MSM before."

- "MSM has given me my life back."

- "Thank God for something natural that relieves my pain without giving me any side effects."

- "Nothing worked for me before this."

- "It's like a miracle."

In this book you will encounter many such remarks from individuals who previously experienced multiple side effects from their medication or whose doctors told them there was nothing more that could be done for them, that they would have to learn to live with the pain.

MSM offers a natural way to reduce pain and inflammation without serious side effects. It may even deliver as much or even more relief as some of the standard painkillers—it just doesn't work as fast. (That's because MSM is not a drug; it is a nutritional supplement.) But you will often begin to experience noticeable easing of pain and discomfort, along with more energy, and in general feel better, within days.

The good news is that MSM is readily available as an inexpensive nutritional supplement in health food stores, drugstores, and through many health practitioners and other accessible outlets. You can purchase it in capsule form to take with a meal as you would any vitamin supplement or use it in crystal form and mix in a drink. You can also buy it as a cream, lotion, or gel and apply it directly to your skin for additional relief from pain and inflammation. You don't need a prescription. It is safe for adults and children alike.

Don't confuse MSM with MSG—monosodium glutamate. MSG is a taste-enhancing agent that frequently causes allergic reactions known as "the Chinese Restaurant syndrome." After many thousands of cases we haven't heard of MSM producing allergic reactions.

In Chapter 3, we tell you how to use MSM and maximize your personal experience of natural pain relief. We give you the practical information on how much to take and answer commonly asked questions about the supplement.

Where Has MSM Been Until Now?

You may be wondering that if MSM is so good why haven't you heard about it before? Until now, there has been little written about it except for a few booklets and articles in nutritional and veterinarian publications. This book is the first comprehensive report on MSM.

Veterinarians have used MSM for more than fifteen years ever since an article on it appeared in an equine journal in the early 1980s. Use by humans goes back nearly twenty years, when one of us (Jacob) began recommending it for patients who came to the world-famous DMSO Clinic at the Oregon Health Sciences University in Portland. MSM was developed from the medical experience with DMSO—dimethyl sulfoxide. You probably have heard of DMSO and may possibly have used it. DMSO is a well-known therapeutic agent derived from trees. MSM is made from DMSO.

DMSO is widely used around the world for relief of arthritis, muscle and skeletal disorders, acute head and spinal cord trauma, athletic injuries, and other conditions. In the U.S., it is approved by the FDA for the treatment of interstitial cystitis, a painful inflammatory disorder of the bladder.

MSM delivers many of the remarkable healing properties of

DMSO—but without the annoying odor of DMSO. Thousands of people, young and old, with various chronic pain conditions, have come to the Portland clinic, often as a last resort because medical treatments weren't working, and have been helped with MSM. It was among such seriously-ill people that the benefits of MSM were first observed.

With interest in alternative medicine and natural remedies soaring, MSM has been brought out of its relatively limited clinical confines into the mainstream of nutritional supplement users. Now its remarkable benefits are being enjoyed by many people interested in natural relief from pain, with no side effects.

MSM is a source of sulfur, a mineral element critical to the normal function and structure of the body. Sulfur is a raw material for the protein and connective tissue that make up our body mass, for enzymes that conduct countless chemical reactions, and for powerful natural compounds that protect us against toxicity and harmful oxidative stress. Sulfur also has a long history of healing but it has been overlooked in our current fascination with vitamins and minerals. When asked to think of minerals important for health, most people know that calcium is good for their bones, that iron is important for their blood, that zinc is needed by the prostate. But rarely does anyone mention sulfur.

In the next chapter we will look at the MSM's "pedigree" and its connection to DMSO and sulfur.

Relief versus Cure

Although much of the scientific fine print relating to MSM's precise healing mechanisms in the body still needs to be determined, we know from clinical experience that it provides major pain relief through the following actions:

- The inhibition of pain impulses along nerve fibers
- Lessening of inflammation
- Increasing of blood supply

- Reduction of muscle spasm
- Softening of scar tissue

In Chapter 4 we spell out in detail MSM's effect on pain in detail and then in Chapter 5 show how it reduces inflammation.

It is our hope that doctors who read this book will consider MSM as an adjunct to their therapies for pain, inflammation, and allergic conditions. MSM can be used with any standard medication without problem. Often patients can reduce and sometimes even discontinue their prescriptions because of MSM's healing effects. But any such modification of medication should be done only under the guidance of a physician. Do not discontinue any prescription without consulting your doctor.

More and more people are using MSM and experiencing healing results similar to what we see in our medical practices. We frequently hear people say, "I'm cured!" Indeed, the effects of MSM are very often quite amazing. It can relieve many painful conditions. Nevertheless, it won't "cure" an illness such as arthritis or lupus. The dictionary defines cure as an elimination of disease. MSM doesn't do that. We don't cure diabetes with insulin. We control it. If we stop the insulin, the diabetic could die. When you think about it, we really don't cure very much at all in medicine and perhaps we shouldn't even use the word. What MSM does is this: It serves as a natural remedy to relieve the pain, inflammation, and many symptoms of illness. Generally, it provides relief for as long as you take it, although sometimes health problems don't return even if you stop taking MSM.

Many people experience rapid relief after starting MSM. We have often heard the statement, "Within a few days my pain was gone." You may indeed experience relief within a few days, but for the very serious chronic conditions we treat in our medical practices we usually see improvement occurring gradually.

Whether relief is fast or slow, this nutritional supplement has real potential to make a significant impact on the quality of life. Some people, of course, may not derive any benefit at all.

How Word Spreads about MSM

Hundreds of millions of dollars are spent by pharmaceutical companies to research and then advertise their patented medical drugs to physicians and consumers. No such bankroll exists for nutritional supplements. That's because nutritional supplements, based on vitamins, minerals, herbs, and natural substances such as MSM, are not patentable.

The major impetus behind MSM's growing popularity is word of mouth. As people experience the healing benefits of MSM, we find they often become enthusiastic emissaries eager to tell family members and friends who have pain problems. One such example is Father Sam, a 46-year-old parish priest in rural Pennsylvania. An avid jogger who has also enjoyed lifting weights in the past, he suffered two sports injuries that left him with a bad shoulder and bad knees.

As he tells it, "A few years ago I began to experience morning pain in both knees, and particularly my right knee, which I had injured during a softball game years before. The pain increased, and with it stiffness and fatigue in my legs. The situation reached the point where my knees were so stiff in the morning that I could hardly walk. In order to go down the steps from the sleeping quarters in our rectory to the main floor, I could move only very slowly, dragging one foot in front of the other."

To go along with his knee pain, Father Sam has a bad shoulder. He overdid it weight lifting about ten years ago.

"I tore tissue in the shoulder or damaged the rotator cuff some way and started to feel the hurt the day after," he says. "The pain lasted for some time and then gradually went away. But three or four years ago the pain returned as arthritis or bursitis connected to the injury. Now it was worse than before, and sometimes the pain would keep me up at night for hours. I would take Tylenol and the pain would go away. But some nights the Tylenol didn't help at all."

Father Sam needed relief. A friend sent him a bottle of MSM and said it might help. It did. Soon after he started taking the MSM, the pain and fatigue in his legs disappeared. The morning stiffness vanished. The pain in his shoulder was gone.

Father Sam is back out in full force on the backroads of central Pennsylvania churning out his four or five miles a day and upward of thirty miles a week, running, as he says, "for the joy of it." He is pain-free as long as he remembers to take the MSM. "When you start to feel better you have a tendency to forget," he says. "If I don't take the MSM for a few days, the pain starts to return. So now I make MSM part of my daily routine—twice a day with orange juice."

Impressed by his positive experience with MSM, Father Sam sent a bottle of MSM capsules to his mother, who suffers from arthritis in the knees. "She had been complaining about the pain for a year," he says. The condition was preventing her from kneeling in church. Because of the pain, she would simply go to her seat without genuflecting. "My mother started taking the pills and also applied an MSM lotion to her knees. Within two or three months, much of her pain was gone and she was able to kneel again in church. She hasn't complained about pain since."

One of the priest's parishioners is Ruth Ann Hubler, the postmistress of Allport, Pennsylvania. She heard him talking one day about how MSM had helped his pain.

"For years I have had arthritis that is particularly bad in my hands," says Hubler. "My fingers were swollen and crooked from the arthritis and hurt from just bending them. I had to have my anniversary ring enlarged so I could wear it. Anytime I bumped my hands into something I would feel the pain. My daily routine of sorting mail into recipients' post office boxes had become very painful because I would always bump my hand against the boxes as I sorted the mail.

"Father Sam suggested I try the same lotion and pills he had used. It was probably a month or so and my hands didn't hurt nearly as much and the swelling had gone down a lot. It's been about a year and now I have no pain at all. The swelling is much less. I have no problems except that now my anniversary ring is loose!"

In Part Two of the book we will describe how MSM relieves common problems such as arthritis, back and muscle pain, headaches, fibromyalgia, and tendinitis. Then, in Part Three, we will discuss MSM's equally amazing effect on allergies.

MSM and Allergies

Many people like Father Sam who take MSM to relieve pain often experience an additional, and unexpected, benefit: relief from allergic symptoms.

"Every year without fail, ever since I was a boy, I endured a perpetually runny nose and nonstop sneezing during pollen season," he says. "It used to be so bad that I had to have allergy shots."

As an adult, he relied on Sinutab, an over-the-counter decongestant for sinus and allergy relief. "I would always be sure to take my Sinutab before Sunday masses," he says. "Sunday morning was of particular concern. I could deal with the allergies more easily during the week because there would be so few people coming to Mass. But on Sundays I have three Masses that are well attended. I didn't want to have a sneezing attack in the middle. Just in case of trouble I had two or three handkerchiefs stuffed in my pockets. The medication usually got me through, but now and then I had to pull out a handkerchief. Without the medication it would have been a disaster."

One evening in the late spring of 1998, Father Sam happened to be watching a television newscast and heard a reporter say the current allergy season was one of the worst in many years. As he heard the report he realized he hadn't been taking his allergy medication and hadn't experienced any symptoms.

"I had totally forgotten about how bad my allergies had been. It dawned on me that here I was in the middle of this bad pollen season not taking the medication and yet I wasn't having any problems," he says. "I was astonished."

Father Sam sailed through the 1998 allergy season on MSM only.

The parish priest's experience is not uncommon. People who take MSM consistently report relief from pain *and* allergies. A mechanic suffered from nose and throat symptoms as a result of pollen that rained down on him from the underside of cars as he worked beneath the vehicles. After taking MSM for a pain problem, he noticed that his pollen allergy had cleared.

MSM offers prompt and powerful relief of pollen allergies, commonly called hay fever—a major seasonal ordeal for some 35 million Americans. MSM may perhaps be as effective as any antihistamine on the market.

Two of the authors of this book (Jacob and Lawrence) have personally experienced the antiallergy benefits of MSM. Both have been plagued by pollen allergies and have taken many medications and natural remedies to counteract allergy symptoms. None has worked as well as MSM.

MSM is a surprising supplement. When you start taking it, you may notice a number of good things happening in your life in addition to pain and allergy relief: more energy; cosmetic benefits such as softer skin, thicker hair, stronger nails; decreased scar tissue; and relief of constipation. In Appendix A we discuss these additional benefits. Finally, in Appendix B, we examine the marketing claims being made about MSM and point out a number of inaccuracies.

In the coming years, with wider and wider usage, more of the healing potential of MSM will be revealed. At this point, based on our clinical experience, we believe that such healing potential may be as great, if not greater, than any other nutritional supplement, and we feel we are only beginning to scratch the surface of its multiple uses. In this book we are covering the major effects known to us. There are no doubt many more benefits that people will discover as they take MSM and use it regularly.

When all the facts are in, and controlled clinical studies are conducted, MSM may become known as one of the great nutritional discoveries of the twentieth century. Still, it is not a panacea. It has its limitations and works at its own speed, which can be quick in some people and slower in others. This book will tell you what to expect from MSM—which is a lot—and what not to expect.

Chapter Two

Roots of MSM—
The DMSO Connection

Dr. Stanley Jacob Explains:

To understand MSM, we need first to understand DMSO. To understand DMSO, we turn the clock back to March 1980, when I appeared on the CBS television show *60 Minutes* with Sandy Sherrick, a southern California housewife. Sherrick had suffered severe chronic whiplash and nerve damage in an automobile accident two years before.

"No pain killer, no therapy, no doctor, it seemed, could help," the show's host Mike Wallace said.

"Oh, the pain was extremely bad. I was to the point where I cried continuously. I did not cook meals. I did not clean. I barely got myself dressed," Sherrick replied.

That was before she came to my Portland clinic for DMSO intravenous treatments—with the cameras of *60 Minutes* rolling to record the progress. By the third day, the program producer observed that Sherrick was feeling better.

"Well, I didn't have to take any more medicine," said Sherrick, who had been taking pain medication continually up until then.

Two months after her treatment, Wallace and his camera crew revisited Sherrick at her home. "The pain is gone," she told them. "The pain is totally, completely gone from my neck."

"You're serious," said Wallace.

"I'm telling the truth, the honest-to-God truth," said Sherrick, and added that she was now doing housework, driving, and in general, functioning quite normally.

Sandy Sherrick, in 1998, is still pain-free, which is unusual when you consider the severity of her injury.

After the *60 Minutes* program, the medical school where my clinic is located was inundated with telephone calls. During the following week, one hundred thousand calls flooded and disabled the school's telephone communication system. The phone in my office rang nonstop. In the year that followed, more than 20 million Americans spent an estimated $1 billion buying DMSO and applying it to their skin for pain relief. They bought it from health food stores, grocery stores, pharmacies, department stores, hobby shops, veterinarians, and even gas stations. Entrepreneurs sold it from home.

The remarkable agent that had attained celebrity status overnight in 1980 was dimethyl sulfoxide—DMSO—a substance I had been working with in my clinic for more than fifteen years.

This naturally occurring sulfur compound was first synthesized a hundred and thirty years ago by a Russian chemist. For nearly a hundred years, it remained a laboratory obscurity. A few chemists published papers on its solvent properties, but it attracted little commercial or industrial interest. A solvent is a compound that dissolves a solid substance into a liquid. Put sugar into coffee, for instance, and the coffee acts as a solvent, dissolving the sugar. Solvents are widely used in industry and chemistry.

In the late 1950s, I was involved in research on kidney transplantation technology at Harvard and the Massachusetts Institute of Technology. I had developed methods to freeze kidneys safely without the organs becoming physically damaged. This was considered a step forward in technology. Until this time, however, the function of the frozen kidneys was still compromised in the process, making them unusable as transplants. Transplantation technology was still rather primitive then.

Around this time I relocated to Portland to head up transplantation research at the University of Oregon Medical School. During my investigations I encountered a scientific paper written by a British scientist named Lovelock about various chemical compounds that permitted freezing red blood cells "alive." One of the compounds was DMSO. I learned that the compound was being produced by Crown-Zellerbach Corporation, a large papermaking concern in adjacent Washington State.

The company made DMSO from lignin, an organic cement-like substance that binds wood fiber together. The first step in the process was extracting dimethyl sulfide (DMS) from the lignin, which was then oxygenated to form DMSO. The company was exploring the solvent potential of DMSO for industrial use.

I contacted Zellerbach and their chemist in charge of DMSO research, Robert Herschler. He provided me with a supply of DMSO and shared his experiences with the compound. We soon began working together in research activities.

Herschler had made the observation that in plants and trees DMSO tended to move through tissues and could carry other materials with it. He was interested in knowing if it could do the same in animals. We found that it did, which made it a quite intriguing compound with the potential to carry medication through the skin and into the body. The DMSO also demonstrated potent pain-reduction and anti-inflammatory properties for people. When applied to the skin over an acute ankle sprain or a burn, for instance, one could see the swelling resolve within an hour.

As research continued, I found that it indeed had many medical properties. DMSO was a diuretic. It had antibacterial effects and even rendered resistant bacteria vulnerable to the same antibiotics to which they had previously been resistant.

With regard to medical transplantation, my original interest in DMSO, the compound turned out to be valuable as a cryoprotective agent—that is, as a preservative for transplantation-bound frozen bone marrow, platelets, embryos, ova, and sperm cells.

Today it is used globally for this purpose. It did not, however, preserve an organ as large as a kidney.

Patients treated in my clinic for pain conditions began spreading the word throughout the Portland area about a new "Oregon wonder drug." The DMSO was impressively relieving the pain of people with severe, unresolved arthritis, bursitis, tendinitis, and many other conditions.

I reported the development for the first time in 1963 at a meeting of the American College of Surgeons. Soon articles began appearing in newspapers, including a front-page article in *The New York Times* describing DMSO as "the most exciting thing in medicine." The uproar was huge. DMSO was suddenly being called a revolution in medicine equivalent to the development of penicillin. Major drug firms came knocking on my door.

The pharmaceutical companies, of course, had their own motives. They were primarily interested in DMSO as a through-the-skin carrier of their own patented medicines. DMSO appeared to be an unparalleled transporter, a highly prized property enabling a drug to enter the bloodstream through the skin and thus bypass the digestive tract where many adverse reactions occur.

By 1965, more than 1,500 studies had been conducted, involving about 100,000 patients, indicating a prescriptive role for a host of problems, primarily musculoskeletal inflammatory conditions. However, during that year, the U.S. Food and Drug Administration (FDA), responsible for approving new drugs, temporarily stopped its consideration of medical uses for DMSO because of the flood of studies it had received and also out of fear of a Thalidomide-like nightmare occurring in the United States. Thalidomide, a sedative drug widely used in Europe, had just been discovered to cause serious deformities of the fetus when taken during pregnancy. The agency was saying "no" to everything, DMSO included. The big companies subsequently lost interest in DMSO.

Without the clout and deep pockets of the pharmaceutical industry, our attempt to win approval for DMSO was an uphill struggle. In 1970, we managed to obtain approval for veterinary usage in the treatment of musculoskeletal disorders. Veterinarians still use it for this purpose on both large and small animals. My hope was that positive results in animals would create momentum for approval for use by humans.

In 1978, the FDA finally approved DMSO as a prescriptive treatment for interstitial cystitis, a painful, inflammatory condition of the bladder affecting a half-million women. To this day, interstitial cystitis remains the only disorder for which DMSO is approved by the FDA, despite numerous congressional hearings recommending wider application. Among athletes, DMSO became particularly popular to speed the healing of typical muscle, ligament, and tendon injuries . . . and is still widely used for that purpose. A special law in the state of Oregon has allowed me to use it for many other conditions—and I have thus been able to help many patients with a variety of severe disorders and musculoskeletal conditions.

In 1973, DMSO became prescriptive in the former Soviet Union. It continues to be prescribed there for an estimated 30 million patients annually with many painful conditions such as lupus, scleroderma, arthritis, and diabetic ulcerations. Globally, DMSO is used in about 125 countries, including Canada, Great Britain, Germany, and Switzerland. I estimate that worldwide it has helped more than a half-billion patients to date. It is safer, less expensive, and at least as effective for a variety of problems for which we presently use other less-effective and more costly treatments. DMSO has been the subject of more than 55,000 studies worldwide.

DMSO is not really a drug. It is more like a multi-functional "therapeutic principle"—an agent with hundreds of properties and applications in the body.

DMSO is safe, a substance of extraordinarily low toxicity, without a single documented death attributed to it. Occasionally a patient is allergic to it. Some individuals who have used industrial-quality DMSO regularly on their skin over a long period of time have reported some minor damage to the skin. The most common side effect, if you want to call it that, is of the nuisance variety—the odor. No matter how DMSO is given—whether intravenously, nasally, orally, instilled into the bladder, under the skin, through the skin, in the muscle, through every conceivable port of entry into the body—it produces a distinctive fish- or oyster-like odor and taste in the mouth. DMSO is widely used internationally to reduce inflammation and carry critical medications through the skin in life-and-death trauma situations. For such short-term applications the odor factor is irrelevant. But used long term for a chronic condition, such as arthritis, the odor becomes bothersome enough so that many people stop taking it.

Enter MSM

In the late 1970s, Robert Herschler suggested studying the properties of DMSO metabolites. Along with other members of the faculty at Oregon Health Sciences University, we began to look at dimethyl sulfone, $DMSO_2$—another scientific name for MSM—which is the major metabolite of DMSO.

When DMSO enters the body approximately 15 percent of it is converted to MSM, its major breakdown component. That means the body attaches an oxygen atom to a portion of the DMSO molecules and they become $DMSO_2$—or MSM. A smaller percentage of DMSO is converted to DMS—dimethyl sulfide. DMS is responsible for producing the odor as well as any skin irritation that may occur. MSM does not produce the DMSO odor. When taken orally or topically, no part of it is converted to DMS.

From prior research, we knew MSM remains in the body longer than DMSO. In a 1967 study, conducted at Merck Sharp & Dohme Research Laboratories, excretion through the urine of orally administered DMSO was complete after 120 hours, "whereas $DMSO_2$ excretion was much more prolonged, lasting until 480 hours or beyond." The researchers suggested that one reason for the longer retention in the body was "possibly more extensive tissue binding." Our observations over the years agree with this assessment. Major DMSO researchers, in fact, have theorized that many of the benefits of DMSO are due to the long-lasting influences of the DMSO fraction converted to MSM.

As I began using MSM with patients, I found it produced

many—but not all—of the DMSO effects. I consider the following to be MSM's most significant actions:

- It is an analgesic. It relieves pain.

- It reduces inflammation.

- It passes through cellular membranes of the body, including the skin.

- It dilates blood vessels (vasodilation) and increases blood flow.

- It is a cholinesterase inhibitor. Cholinsterase is an enzyme that stops excessive passage of nerve impulses from one nerve cell to another. I have seen MSM provide swift relief of constipation associated with aging. By blocking the action of cholinesterase, MSM helps restore normal bowel activity (peristalsis).

- It reduces muscle spasm. Injury or inflammation commonly cause spasm in a muscle or group of muscles. Spasm involves a sudden contraction, which is followed by pain and interference with function. Spasm can be felt by a physician's touch or measured with electromyography. If you apply an MSM gel or cream to an affected area and then feel the muscle again later, or measure it electrically, the muscle is looser, the area less tender. MSM taken orally produces a muscle-relaxing effect.

- It alters the crosslinking process in collagen, thus reducing scar tissue. Crosslinking is the process in which new structural proteins are knitted to existing healthy tissue at the sites of surgical incisions or traumatic damage in the body.

- It has antiparasitic properties, particularly for giardia, a protozoan parasite that causes diarrhea.

- It has an immune normalizing effect, as observed in some autoimmune diseases such as rheumatoid arthritis, lupus, and scleroderma.

One of the factors that set both DMSO and MSM apart is that they are small molecules. DMSO tips the scales at a molecular weight of 78; MSM, 94. By chemistry standards, they are feather-weight molecules. They mimic water in this respect. Water has a very low molecular weight and passes through tissue. DMSO and MSM pass through the skin and into the tissue below. Just like DMSO, MSM is very useful when employed as a topical gel, cream, or lotion to help in the relief of local pain and inflammation. Unlike DMSO, however, MSM cannot transport medication with it.

Another difference between the two compounds is that DMSO is a proven and powerful free-radical scavenger, that is, an antioxidant, whereas MSM's antioxidant significance at this point is unclear. Free radicals are unstable molecular fragments that launch an oxidative attack on DNA, cell membranes, enzymes, and proteins, disrupting normal cellular activities and trigger the inflammatory process. Such cumulative oxidative damage is similar to the rusting of metal and contributes to premature aging and the development of serious disease. Every disease known to medical science is associated with an increased activity of free radicals.

One of the first things we set out to learn about MSM was its safety. In long-term toxicity trials with laboratory animals we found no toxic effects with oral doses of 8 grams per kilogram (2.2 pounds) of body weight. Most people take from 2 to 8 grams total as a daily supplement.

To determine the lethal dose of MSM, or of any substance, we used a standard test known as LD-50. LD stands for lethal dose. The number 50 refers to the amount of the substance required that would result in the death of half the number of laboratory animals used in the test. For MSM, the findings determined that the LD-50 was more than 20 grams for each kilogram of body weight. To put that into perspective, the LD-50 of common table salt you use for cooking is 2.5 to 3 grams per kilogram of weight. MSM thus rates as one of the least toxic substances in biology and medicine. It compares to water, which has an LD-50 rating also greater than 20 grams per kilogram of weight.

In follow-up experiments with human volunteers, we found

no toxic effects at intake levels of up to 1 gram per kilogram of body weight per day for 30 days. That means about 68 grams for an average 150-pound person. A few patients have taken more than 100 grams orally of MSM daily without any side effects. But these were extremely unusual cases involving very sick patients under my personal care. Do not take that much on your own. Please refer to Chapter 3 for details on how much MSM to take.

In a paper presented to the New York Academy of Sciences in 1982, Herschler and I described the actions, benefits, and nontoxicity of MSM for the first time. In the ensuing years, I continued to use MSM with great success in my clinic and found that it was well-tolerated and provided wonderful relief for people with pain, inflammation, constipation, and other common problems. Veterinarians became interested in MSM and found it beneficial for horses and dogs suffering from arthritis and lameness. Many people, seeing the benefits for their animals, started buying MSM from veterinarians and tack shops and using it themselves. Word spread over the years—first from patients and then from animal owners. Finally, with the explosion of interest in alternative medicine and natural remedies that has occurred during this decade, a number of manufacturers saw the promise of MSM as a nutritional supplement and began marketing it. Now, MSM has the potential to join the growing array of natural substances such as melatonin and St. John's Wort that can be used by a broad number of people to reduce common health problems.

MSM in Nature

In its natural state MSM is an inconspicuous sulfur molecule found in the atmosphere, in plants, animals, and the human body. Chemically, it consists of two hydrocarbon units (groups of hydrogen and carbon atoms) attached to a unit with one sulfur and two oxygen atoms. The molecule is one-third sulfur by weight.

Atmospheric chemists describe the molecule as a minor oxidation product in an oceanic sulfur cycle that begins with marine algae. These ocean organisms, called phytoplankton, release sulfur compounds known as dimethylsulfonium salts. The salts, in turn, are transformed in the ocean water into a volatile compound—dimethylsulfide (DMS)—which escapes as a gas from watery depths and rises into the atmosphere. There, the DMS undergoes photochemical oxidation and is converted to sulfur compounds, mostly sulfates, and, in part, to $DMSO_2$ (MSM) as well as dimethyl sulfoxide (DMSO), the closest relative of MSM. These compounds are absorbed in tiny droplets called aerosols that float around the atmosphere and are returned to the surface of the ocean with rainwater.

On land, a number of scientific analyses over the years have found MSM present naturally in animal tissue, food, and in the human body. Researchers first discovered the molecule more than fifty years ago in the blood, adrenal glands, and milk of cows. It was also found to be present in horses and rabbits and assumably is there in other species.

Later, in a 1982 analysis by the Crown-Zellerbach Company, milk was found to contain between 2 and 6 parts per million of MSM. That may not seem like much but the quantity is higher than the level of some other better-known minerals, such as manganese and selenium. Zinc, by comparison, weighs in at 8.6 parts per million in milk. Coffee contains about 1.5 parts of MSM per million, and tea somewhat less. Green vegetables and other foods have small traces of MSM.

MSM's presence in the human body was first reported during the 1960s, when a laboratory analysis of the urine of men, women, and children found that 4 to 11 milligrams of MSM was excreted over a twenty-four-hour period. Then in the late 1980s, a researcher at a major German pharmaceutical company found that MSM is present in human plasma. Plasma is the liquid part of blood. Through a gas chromatography technique, W. Martin of Pharmakin Gmbh of Ulm detected a "significant concentration" of MSM among the one hundred samples of plasma he examined. He found the equivalent of about 4 milligrams of MSM in the plasma of an average-size adult.

So far, researchers have not adequately been able to explain the presence of MSM other than that it comes from food sources and/or is the result of a natural chain of biochemical reactions. Its precise role is not known.

Through other research we have learned that MSM is utilized inside the body. This was first demonstrated in animal studies conducted by Virginia Richmond of the Pacific Northwest Research Foundation in Seattle and reported in the journal *Life Sciences* in 1986. In her experiments, she fed MSM with radioactive sulfur in it to guinea pigs. Radioactively "labeled" elements are used in scientific research to track the utilization of substances in the body. A subsequent analysis of serum proteins revealed that a small amount of the MSM sulfur had been taken up by two of the body's sulfur amino acids, methionine and cysteine.

Three studies conducted with laboratory mice at the Oregon Health Sciences University and Ohio State University showed that supplemental MSM was absorbed by laboratory mice and significantly delayed the onset of cancer created under experimental conditions. Other promising animal studies suggested that MSM may improve autoimmune diseases in which the body's own immune system becomes deranged and starts to attack its own tissue. Rheumatoid arthritis and lupus are two of the better-known autoimmune diseases. In these experiments, researchers found they could substantially prolong the lifespan of certain breeds of mice prone to such abnormalities by adding MSM to their drinking water. The rodents used in these trials were particularly susceptible to autoimmune illness.

As practicing physicians, our ability to personally conduct rigorous scientific research is limited. Our focus is treating patients. Yet when each of us carried out independent studies in our individual clinics on patients suffering from the severe pain of degenerative arthritis, we reached the same conclusion— pronounced relief of pain.

These, and other results we have seen among patients, are impressive. The studies to date are tantalizing but preliminary. More are needed. Hopefully, this book will promote further research necessary to understand better this unique and natural substance that perpetuates a long sulfur healing tradition.

Sulfur in Your Body and in the Healing Tradition

A "healing" of sorts occurred in biblical times when brimstone, the old name for sulfur, rained down from heaven to extinguish the sin spots of Sodom and Gomorrah. What form of brimstone rained down nobody knows, but we do know that sulfur spews out of volcanoes and coal furnaces to pollute the air as sulfur dioxide. It is one of the very few minerals that are combustible.

Four thousand years ago, the Egyptians burned the yellow powder of sulfur to ward off bad spirits. Throughout the ages since, man has put sulfur to varied but history-altering use. The Chinese discovered gunpowder by mixing sulfur and saltpeter, thus opening a new dimension in our ability to kill one another.

In Latin, it was called *sol ferrein*, meaning "carrying the sun," a reference to the yellow color of the mineral—a reflection of the sun.

In our modern age, sulfur compounds have made huge economic contributions. As Ryan Huxtable of the University of Arizona noted in his 1986 textbook *Biochemistry of Sulfur* (Plenum Press), "The industrialized world rolls on tires vulcanized with sulfur and more sulfuric acid is manufactured than any other chemical." Sulfur compounds are utilized for fertilizers, fungicides, fumigants, cellophane, rayon, nylon fibers, textiles, dyes, gasoline, steel, pulp for paper and bleaching of dried fruits, just to name a few of its many applications.

In plants, sulfur is found mostly in protein and also in compounds that give certain plants their famous odors—onions, garlic, horseradish, and cabbage, for instance. Sulfur, in fact, is fairly synonymous with smells.

"Some, such as those (compounds) present in skunk odor and flatulence, we find repellent," wrote Huxtable. "Others, such as those found in truffles, coffee and asparagus, the majority of us find attractive. Others, again, exemplified by the sulfur-containing constituents of garlic and onions, we may at times find attractive, and on other occasions, distasteful." The connection of sulfur with odors and volcanoes, adds Huxtable, has bestowed the mineral with a "Mephistophelean reputation that masks its fundamental importance in biological processes."

Sulfur is not just around us, but inside us as well. Our body puts sulfur to great use. It's an integral part of what makes us and what makes us tick. Sulfur is the eighth most abundant element in all living organisms. In our bodies, it forms part of virtually all tissues, especially those highest in protein, such as red blood cells, muscles, skin, and hair.

Ever burned a strand of hair in an open flame and noticed the odor? That's the smell of sulfur. Your hair contains a lot of sulfur. So do your nails and skin. One of the most frequent comments we hear from people, particularly women who are taking MSM, is that their hair and nails have become stronger. This is yet another indication that the sulfur in MSM is biologically active and is being absorbed and utilized by the body.

When you weigh yourself, about 1 percent of the number you read on the scale is sulfur. In all fairness, if you're overweight, don't blame it on sulfur. Sulfur isn't fattening. Neither is MSM, we should hasten to add.

Sulfur is a major ingredient of important amino acids—the building blocks of proteins. Proteins are the primary constituents of enzymes, hormones, antibodies, and the countless biochemical activities continually going on in the body. Proteins also provide the structural raw material of muscles, bones, hair, teeth, blood, brains, skin, and the other organs of the body. If you don't get enough protein, you suffer all over. In children, deficiency retards growth. In adults, it shows up as chronic fatigue, mental depression, weakness, poor resistance to infection, and slow healing from wounds or disease.

Molecules of protein are comprised of twenty-four amino acids, and because of the many ways these amino acids can combine to form a protein, there are endless numbers of different proteins. Among the amino acids is a group known as the sulfur amino acids, which means that these compounds contain sulfur. Foremost among them are methionine and cysteine.

Methionine is an essential amino acid, meaning you must get

it in the food you eat. Your body doesn't make it, as it does many other amino acids. Methionine has several main roles. Primary among them is methylation, a fundamental process that triggers biochemical changes throughout the body, altering the structure and function of hormones as well as other proteins and amino acids.

Cysteine is not an essential amino acid. Your body makes it from methionine. But it performs big chores in the body, including protection of sensitive tissue from excess oxidation that causes disease and premature aging. Cysteine is the key ingredient in glutathione, a molecular "superman" found in virtually all living cells. It is a primary antioxidant and detoxifying agent in the body. Among other things, it helps the body rid itself of some carcinogens and hazardous chemicals.

The body uses methionine and cysteine also to form such essential compounds as insulin, which regulates carbohydrate metabolism, and heparin, an anticoagulant. Sulfur amino acids are also involved as essential players in the energy metabolism that takes place in the mitochondria—the "power plants" inside every cell. Sulfur is also found in thiamine and biotin. These two important B complex vitamins are also essential for energy production. Sulfur plays an important role in healthy skin, cartilage, and connective tissue and is vital to healing wounds. Sulfate, a more oxidized form of sulfur, is used by the liver to detoxify substances, make them more water-soluble, and prepare them biochemically for excretion by the kidneys.

Thus, sulfur participates in many basic structural and functional aspects of your being. More than just a raw material, it contributes to the process of life. It is involved in the building up of our body substance, the energy that sustains our physical activity, and the neutralization of oxidants and toxins that can destroy our health from within.

From a healing perspective, there is something very special about sulfur. No matter where you travel—near or far—chances are you'll find a sulfur hot spring with a healing tradition or mystique attached to it.

In ancient times, Agamemnon, leader of the Greek states in

the Trojan Wars, is said to have brought his wounded soldiers to the Balcova hot springs near Izmir, in Turkey. To this day, the "Baths of Agamemnon," as they are called, are recommended for rheumatic diseases, digestive disorders, and post-operative conditions.

Mozart and Beethoven frequented a sulfur spring at Baden, near Vienna. In Italy, the elegant Salsomaggiore sulfur baths have attracted the likes of the wife of Napoleon I, Enrico Caruso, and Luciano Pavarotti.

On St. Lucia in the West Indies, simmering sulfur water that "fills the air with an odor of rotting eggs" cascades down from Soufrière volcano into baths below. Louis XVI, it is said, recommended the restorative waters to rejuvenate his tired troops.

In Japan, the Harazuru Sulfur Springs in Fukuoka Prefecture is an all-year facility "which works well for rheumatism and neuralgia," according to the local promoters.

Hot Springs, Montana, beckons visitors to its healing "Big Medicine" waters, discovered by Native American tribes, and said to produce relaxation and relief from arthritis, skin diseases, stomach ulcers, high blood pressure, and many other conditions.

The medical literature contains past references to the use of sulfur-rich baths for healing purposes, particularly arthritis. Although sulfur baths still attract many patients, their popularity as a primary curative treatment has waned with the advent of modern medical methods.

In the ageless healing tradition of sulfur, one cannot ignore garlic, perhaps the most famous—and oldest—of all sulfur medicinals. John Heinerman, Ph.D., in his book *The Healing Benefits of Garlic* (Keats Publishing), traces the use of garlic for healing back some 4,300 years to the Sumerian civilization of the Euphrates River Valley—now Iraq. According to Sumerian tablets excavated in the 1930s, garlic was used by these ancient people for fevers, loose bowels, inflammation, strained muscles, pulled ligaments, parasites, and as a general tonic. Many ancient cultures, Heinerman wrote, "considered garlic to be one of the most important spices for feeding and healing the human body."

In a much later era, Louis Pasteur discovered that garlic

destroyed harmful bacteria. And still later, Albert Schweitzer used garlic compounds to treat amoebic dysentery. Researchers have found at least 100 sulfur compounds in garlic and have validated many of its folk medicine applications.

Organic sulfur compounds are not exclusive to garlic. You can, as a matter of fact, tell which foods and herbs are high in sulfur content by their odor. "Foods that have a distinct smell when they're cooked (such as cabbage), or make your eyes water when cut (such as onions), or grab your taste buds by their roots with an unmistakable pungency (like horseradish), have an abundance of sulfur," wrote Heinerman. Interestingly, he noted that foods like cabbage, kale, kohlrabi, Brussels sprouts, mustard greens, watercress, leeks, onion, radish, cauliflower, and horseradish—all sulfur-bearing foods—have properties that have been demonstrated in scientific studies to inhibit certain types of experimentally induced cancers.

"The purifying and beneficial properties of sulfur have been known for millennia," wrote Stephen C. Mitchell, M.D., editor of *Biological Interactions of Sulfur Compounds* (Taylor & Francis), and "probably a quarter of pharmaceutical products presently used contain sulfur." Among the most famous of them are penicillin and cephalosporin antibiotics.

Are You Sulfur— or MSM—Deficient?

Many users of MSM believe the supplement remedies a sulfur deficiency in the body. Sulfur is a mineral nutrient found in food, and minerals are frequently deficient in the Western diet with serious consequences to health. Magnesium and zinc are two leading examples of commonly deficient minerals. Unlike magnesium and zinc, for which there are recognized daily intake standards, no such yardstick exists for sulfur intake.

From a nutritional standpoint, sulfur—like Rodney Dangerfield—receives little respect. Although it is clearly necessary for health, sulfur per se is not regarded as an essential nutritional element. The U.S. Academy of Sciences' Food and Nutrition Board, which creates the recommended daily allowance for nutrients—the suggested amount we should eat in order to maintain health—doesn't include sulfur in its considerations. By comparison, recommendations exist for a number of other mineral nutrients, such as calcium, potassium, magnesium, and zinc. Physicians know that you need a certain level of these minerals in your diet and can often trace health problems to low intakes.

The late Carl Pfeiffer, Ph.D., M.D., a world-renowned expert on nutritional medicine, once described sulfur as "the forgotten essential element."

The cause of sulfur neglect is anchored to the widespread assumption that a person's sulfur requirement is met when protein intake is adequate. When not enough protein is ingested, deficiency diseases develop—the kind you see associated with starvation in Africa, for instances, where bodies literally fall apart.

In our typical Western diet, adequate protein usually isn't a problem. If anything, nutritionists say, we may eat too much protein. The elderly, however, may not consume enough protein, according to a recent study in the *Journal of Clinical Investigation*. Researchers at the University of Texas suggest that the loss of muscle mass associated with aging may be avoided if adequate protein is eaten. Muscle atrophy in the elderly leads to a reduction in performance, increased risk of falls, and a heightened susceptibility to bone fractures.

Two important constituents of protein, the amino acids methionine and cysteine, provide us with a paramount source of sulfur. These aminos are present in the animal protein sources of meat, fish, eggs, and dairy products. From the plant world, proteins from garlic, onions, asparagus, avocados, beans, peas, cabbage, Brussels sprouts, broccoli, cauliflower, mustard, horseradish, and sunflower seeds are also sulfur bearers. And, yes, even chocolate has a bit. The cruciferous vegetables—such as cabbage, Brussels sprouts, broccoli, and cauliflower—also contain other sulfur compounds not related to amino acids that have been identified as important contributors to the body's natural detoxification processes.

Given the range of food choices, it appears understandable why a sulfur deficiency is assumed to be nonexistent. Beyond the assumption, however, there is little evidence. Medical science knows a good deal about deficiencies of many vitamins and minerals, but not about sulfur.

One sulfur researcher at a major university put it this way: "People look so little at sulfur nutritionally because it is so well known that sulfur-containing proteins, which are in the foods we eat, must be present in plants or else the plants don't grow. When we meet our protein requirements we have enough sulfur produced through the breakdown of the protein to obtain the body's sulfur needs. Basically, anything we eat with protein in it is going to have sulfur amino acids, primarily methionine and cysteine."

Asked about sulfur deficiency in the population, a spokeswoman at the U.S. Department of Agriculture Nutrient Data Laboratory simply said, "Sulfur isn't something we compile data on. We don't list the sulfur content of foods. It's not on our radar screen." Another government nutrition official said she doesn't remember "ever" seeing a study on sulfur. "We look at a lot of minerals, including tin and even arsenic," she said. "But sulfur isn't even among them."

Americans are notoriously deficient in many important nutrients because of our poor eating habits, which has a lot to do with our poor health statistics. A 1996 University of San Francisco study that made nationwide headlines concluded that nearly 100 million of us—40 per cent of the population—are afflicted with some form of chronic ailment. Could there be an unrecognized sulfur deficiency—marginal enough to contribute to this bleak statistic? Nobody has a real answer yet.

Melvyn R. Werbach, M.D., a well-known medical researcher and author of *Nutritional Influences on Illness* (Third Line Press), questions assumptions being made about adequacies of sulfur or any nutrient. "I have been surprised in my research to find so little information about sulfur," he says. "There are big, big holes in our knowledge about this mineral nutrient. How do we really know there isn't a sulfur deficiency?"

Muddled Methionine

The food choices that many of us make—nutrient-poor diets heavy in processed, devitalized foods—contribute to self-inflicted deficiencies and imbalances of many different vitamins, minerals, and amino acids. Nutritional surveys continually show vast numbers of Americans with low or suboptimal intakes of essential nutrients, levels that experts such as Harvard nutritional researchers Meir Stampfer and Walter Willett say are "strongly . . . associated with serious health consequences."

Methionine, as we have seen earlier, is an essential sulfur amino acid we must obtain from our diet. The body processes methionine into other important sulfur amino acids—cysteine, cystine, and taurine, plus countless hormones and structural proteins. While medical science recognizes the existence of certain inherited disorders of amino acid and sulfur metabolism, the major problems related to methionine probably lie elsewhere: a lack of good vitamins and minerals—the nutritional co-factors—needed to process methionine properly. Minerals such as magnesium and zinc, as well as the B-complex vitamins B_6 and folic acid are all commonly deficient in the average diet.

In the case of a B_6 and folic acid shortage, the results can be catastrophic: The liver is unable to properly process methionine. In a complex biochemical sequence, this shortage causes a rise in the level of homocysteine, a toxic amino acid. Elevated homocysteine has been found to trigger vascular disease that takes the lives of nearly a million Americans a year and affects more than 57 million individuals. Homocysteine is being increasingly seen as a more significant heart attack and stroke risk factor than cholesterol. We don't eat enough whole grains, fruits, and vegetables—excellent sources of vitamin B_6 and folic acid. Instead, we eat enormous amounts of refined, denuded grains, and consume considerable quantities of sugar-laden foods and animal protein, which deplete the body of B complex vitamins, particularly B_6.

Other reasons for problems with methionine include the aging process. Nutrient levels tend to decline with age as the body becomes less efficient. We know that many vitamins and minerals—including B_6 and folic acid—are present in lower quantities in the elderly than in younger people. The level of digestive enzymes, necessary for proper protein and methionine breakdown, also decline with age.

In addition to these considerations, there is evidence associating abnormalities or low levels of sulfur-bearing amino acids in patients with a variety of disorders. Such evidence appeared in an issue on sulfur (August 1997) in *The Moss Nutrition Report,* a nationally circulated newsletter written by Jeffrey Moss, D.D.S., a Massachusetts-based nutritional researcher. Moss cited the following references, among others:

- In a textbook on amino acid metabolism, Vernon R. Young and Antoine E. El-Khoury of the Massachusetts Institute of Technology question "the prevailing dogma . . . (that) the physiological requirements for the sulfur amino acids can be fully met through a generous intake of methionine alone," and particularly during situations of severe physical trauma and stress.

- An analysis of nutritional and metabolic data by Jon Pangborn, Ph.D., a well-known nutritional biochemist affiliated with the Great Smokies Diagnostic Laboratories in Asheville, North Carolina, found that the metabolism of methionine is the "most frequently impaired or disordered amino acid" among 1,500 individuals with food and chemical intolerances, degenerative diseases, neuromuscular dysfunction, and mental diseases.

"These findings do not prove or disprove nutritional deficiency," wrote Moss. "However, they lend strong support to the assumption that methionine metabolism is imbalanced in sick people."

In his book *Mental and Elemental Nutrients* (Keats Publishing), Carl Pfeiffer, Ph.D., M.D., looked back to the nineteenth century where elemental sulfur was used to treat many disorders because no better remedies were available. "If these uses are reviewed with the thought that sulfur deficiency may perhaps occur in man as well as in animals, then some of the old uses of sulfur make good sense," he wrote.

MSM, as you will read later in this book, reduces many of the symptoms associated with the conditions just mentioned. In addition to its DMSO-related properties, it may play a role in correcting sulfur amino acid abnormalities and possible sulfur deficiencies. We know from animal studies that a small amount of sulfur from MSM supplementation enters into methionine and cysteine in the body. This utilization could fortify these crucial amino acids.

Do people in a health crisis or recovering from trauma, have an increased demand for more sulfur? We know that a body under physiologic stress has an increased demand for more nutrients. Does that include an increased need for sulfur?

Does the sulfur payload of MSM strengthen the body's ability to carry out critical detoxification and tissue-building activities in times of physical stress?

Can an MSM supplement come in, like a white knight, and cover these bases?

At this point in time, we have many questions but not all the answers. We know from our clinical observations that MSM helps reduce pain, inflammation, and other symptoms, and it accelerates healing without adverse side effects. What we need are additional scientific studies to answer many important issues, hitherto largely neglected, about the role of sulfur in health and illness.

A New Generation of Awareness, a New Breed of Nutrients

Our modern medical system performs brilliantly in the area of emergency medicine, acute care treatment, and sophisticated surgical procedures. Yet the system often falls short in dealing with chronic ailments. Many of the approved treatments, procedures, and drugs cause substantial—and even deadly—new symptoms. Despite the highest medical costs in the world, we have some of the worst health statistics of all industrialized countries. In a 1993 ranking of health among the developed nations, the World Health Organization (WHO) listed the U.S. as eighteenth!

Many patients do not benefit from standard medical treatments and go elsewhere for relief, to so-called alternative practitioners, even if they have to pay out of their own pockets. In 1990, one-third of Americans visited an alternative doctor, spending about $14 billion out of their own pockets for 425 million office visits not covered by conventional health plans, according to a 1993 *New England Journal of Medicine* study that put real numbers on a growing consumer trend for the first time.

In a 1998 Standford University study published in the *Journal of the American Medical Association,* 40 percent of more than one thousand randomly selected people around the U.S. said they used some form of alternative health care during the previous year. The most frequently cited health problem treated with alternative therapy, the report said, was chronic pain (37 percent).

This consumer trend has rocked the medical establishment. Increasing numbers of medical schools are offering courses in alternative practices. Hospitals and medical centers are opening wings to deliver alternative treatments. Late in 1998, the *Journal of the American Medical Association* devoted an entire issue to studies evaluating alternative treatments. According to a 1998 *Los Angeles Times* series, thirty major insurers are now covering more than one form of alternative medicine.

Within this overall medical shift a new attitude has developed toward nutritional supplements. Prior to 1990, vitamins and minerals were viewed narrowly by most physicians as necessary elements contained in food that prevented nutritional deficiency states such as scurvy, beriberi, rickets, and pellagra. The prevailing attitude held that supplementation was unnecessary because a balanced diet was supposed to provide all the good nutrition our bodies needed. For decades, only a small minority of nutritionally oriented physicians advocated supplements as a potent, safe, and inexpensive way to help treat illness and create optimum health.

Current nutritional research has weakened the conventional viewpoint and supported the minority idea. For one thing, nutritionists acknowledge that huge numbers of people fail to eat anything resembling a balanced or nutritionally sound diet. In addition, many studies now show that individual nutrients at doses higher than those usually present in the diet can have a profound preventive and therapeutic impact against serious diseases. Massive consumer interest and an avalanche of scientific discoveries about vitamin, mineral, amino acid, herbal, and phytochemical (natural plant compounds) supplementation in recent years are causing physicians to take a broader look at the health-promoting and cost-reducing potential that these natural substances offer.

Research has demonstrated, for instance, that vitamin E supplementation combats arterial plaque formation and enhances immune function. Contemporary studies have backed the clinical observations of Canadian physicians Wilfrid and Evan Shute, first made more than fifty years ago, that vitamin E helped ailing hearts. While the medical community shunned the Shute brothers, it was their persistent reporting of positive, and often dramatic experiences with patients, that led to the popularity of vitamin E today.

At a landmark 1992 symposium sponsored by the New York Academy of Science, researchers presented many new findings on the beneficial effects of vitamins and minerals against cancer, heart disease, and other illnesses. The symposium was called "Beyond Deficiency: New Views on the Function and Health Effects of Vitamins." *Medical World News,* a periodical read by many doctors, led off its January 1993 issue with an article entitled "Vitamins: Emerging as Disease Fighters, Not Just Supplements." The article said that new studies on the role of vitamins are shifting the foundations of nutrition research, policy, and public health in this country.

A whole new era appears to be dawning where physicians will be guided in their treatment of illness by integrative methods combining the best of pharmaceutical, surgical, and natural tools available to them. A new breed of food-based substances and natural compounds has emerged as exciting new nutritional supplements to participate in this new healing age. MSM is one of them.

Chapter Three

How to Take MSM

MSM is a nutritional supplement with many nurturing and health-enhancing properties. If you are under treatment for any condition that is mentioned in this book, we recommend that you bring our observations to your physician's attention and obtain his or her professional opinion regarding your use of the supplement. In many instances, MSM's beneficial effects on the body permit a reduction in prescriptive medication, which, in turn, may reduce side effects.

Please keep your doctor informed. Do not reduce medication on your own.

Q: *What are the available forms of MSM?*
A: The general use of MSM is either orally, as capsules or crystals, or applied topically to the skin as a lotion, cream, or gel.

Q: *What is the best form of MSM?*
A: You should take whatever form is most convenient for you. If you are taking 2 or 3 grams a day or less, the capsules may be the most convenient. For higher doses, you may like to use MSM

crystals and mix them into water, juice, or any nonalcoholic beverage, including coffee or tea.

A level measured pharmacist's teaspoon holds about 4 grams, or 4,000 milligrams of MSM crystals. A level kitchen teaspoon, somewhat larger, will hold about 5 grams (5,000 milligrams). The crystals have a bitter taste.

Q: *How much MSM should I take?*

A: Whether you're taking a medication or a nutritional supplement, you should always take the least possible amount that gives you the benefit you desire. This same idea applies to MSM. More is not necessarily better.

Each of us are unique individuals with different genetic makeup, sizes, hormones, tolerances, energy, resistance, and levels of health or illness. Even if two people have the same type and severity of disease, each brings into play a different set of strengths and weaknesses with which to counteract it.

Because we are so different, our bodies also respond somewhat differently to medication. One aspirin may work for your headache but your brother with the same headache may need two. The same is true of natural remedies and nutritional supplements. One gram of MSM may give you a shot of energy but your brother may need five grams to feel the same effect.

Over the years, thousands of patients have experienced healing benefits by taking 2 to 8 grams (2,000 to 8,000 milligrams) of MSM a day, the amount depending on their gastrointestinal (or GI) tolerance and their condition.

For general maintenance and health, a dosage of around 2 grams (2,000 milligrams) or less is usually adequate.

Higher doses are typically necessary to experience therapeutic effects. You may need 3 to 4 grams of MSM a day to control your allergic symptoms of sneezing, runny nose, and burning eyes during pollen season.

For severe, deep-seated conditions, you will probably need higher doses, and sometimes much higher, to experience relief. We have used extremely large doses in the treatment of extraordinary cases. We have recommended 40 or 60 grams and up in incremental daily doses for severe conditions, but in these instances patients were under our personal supervision.

It is our opinion that the higher the dose you can take without developing an upset stomach the quicker you will experience a healing response and the fewer symptomatic recurrences you will have. If you don't see a response, increase your dosage slowly.

Start low. Work up slowly. That's our general recommendation. Build up to an optimum dose perhaps over a two- or three-week period. Many people start off with 2 grams a day and increase another gram or two after several days. If you wish to go higher, raise your dose again by a similar amount several days later.

As you raise the level of MSM it is a good idea to divide the doses during the day. That helps your body become accustomed to the MSM.

This is not a cookbook. Dosages are not carved in stone. The recommendations we make are based on years of clinical experience. Just remember the individuality principle.

Q: *What if I take too much MSM?*
A: If you overdo it, you may develop minor gastrointestinal discomfort or more frequent stools. Just cut back if that happens.

Taking MSM in two or three doses over the day reduces the possibility of a GI reaction. Divided doses are recommended in particular for people taking larger quantities of MSM.

We have heard that some athletes and bodybuilders involved in high-intensity training start with relatively high levels of MSM to increase stamina and reduce muscle soreness. Some take 5 or more grams before and after workouts right from the start. We have been told that a number of them have experienced headaches or GI reactions in the beginning. Our recommendation for athletes and nonathletes alike is always to start low and build up slowly.

For pain and inflammatory conditions, and musculo-skeletal problems, we generally recommend the "double-barreled approach"—MSM orally and topically. Topically means applying an MSM gel or lotion to the affected area.

Q: *Should I take MSM on an empty stomach or with meals?*

A: Although many people take it on an empty stomach, it is probably best to have some food in the stomach. Taking it during or after meals minimizes the chance of developing the possibility of minor gastrointestinal upset when you first start using it.

As a general rule, don't take MSM close to bedtime. It might keep you awake. MSM has the tendency to increase your energy level.

Q: *How fast does MSM work?*

A: There is no way to predict your response because every situation is different. Benefits can occur immediately, within days, or they can take much longer. Some people start to notice an appreciable decrease in pain the day after starting the supplement. For others, noticeable improvement may take months.

Q: *How safe is MSM?*

A: The overwhelming majority of people have no problem with MSM. It is extremely safe. We haven't heard of any serious side effects to date. Thousands of patients have taken two grams and more daily of MSM for many months and years with no serious side effects.

Nevertheless, it should be pointed out that MSM is a biologically active substance. It has pharmacologic activity, meaning it can produce effects in the body. Such effects are described in this book and are virtually of a positive nature. Still, any agent with pharmacologic activity also has the potential for side effects.

Any substance on the planet, including water, has the potential to cause a reaction in some person somewhere. If you are a hypersensitive individual and have any doubts about using this supplement, consult with your physician first.

As already stated, taking too large a dose at one time for your particular constitution could cause some minor gastrointestinal upset, increased stool, or minimal abdominal cramping. If this occurs, reduce the level of MSM. That should take care of the discomfort.

Some people who might benefit the most from higher doses may not be able to reach their optimum level because of GI intolerance. After reducing the dosage to a level that you tolerate, you can try very slowly raising it again. However, if your body says "that's it," then listen. Your body knows best.

Experience over the years suggests that MSM may have a similar dosage characteristic as vitamin C. By that we mean that if the body has a greater need for it there is a greater tolerance for higher doses.

It is well known that the sicker you are, the more vitamin C your body utilizes and tolerates. As an example, if you were to take 5 grams of vitamin C you might get temporary diarrhea. That is the major side effect of taking too much vitamin C. If you have a heavy cold or flu, you might be able to take 20 grams, or even much more in a very severe situation, without incurring any diarrhea.

Physicians familiar with vitamin C therapeutics refer to this as bowel tolerance. The sicker you are, the more your body needs, and the more you tolerate. Once you are healthy again, your body would not need the high level of the vitamin, and large doses would once again cause diarrhea. It is just below these bowel tolerance levels, the experts say, that vitamin C has its most powerful therapeutic effect.

There have been accounts in the medical literature of occasional minor skin rashes associated with DMSO. Because MSM is a related substance, the potential for a similar reaction also exists. Again, reducing dosage usually takes care of the problem. If it does not, than stop the MSM and try to resume it again in a few days but at a reduced level. If you develop a rash again, you should probably discontinue taking the supplement.

Temporary minor headaches may occasionally occur in the very beginning if a person starts at too high a level. For this reason we always recommend starting on a low dosage and increasing slowly.

Q: *If I take too much MSM could it kill me?*

A: In Chapter 2 we talked about the safety of MSM. We have studied the safety issue in a number of experiments, one of which is a standard scientific test known as LD-50. This test determines how much of any given substance is lethal to laboratory animals. MSM was shown to have one-seventh the "toxicity" of common table salt. That means it is very safe and comparable, we believe, to water. In more than twenty years of MSM usage, we have never heard that it caused any serious reactions.

Q: *Can I take MSM indefinitely?*

A: We have patients who have taken MSM for nearly twenty years. One of our daughters has been taking MSM for eighteen years. She is now in her early twenties. We gave it to her because we feel it has many protective benefits, including strengthening the immune system. There is no scientific evidence for that, but people who take it regularly appear to have fewer colds and viral infections.

One of us (Jacob) has been taking MSM for many years.

We have found that many people derive benefits from MSM only as long as they continue to take it. Once the supplement is discontinued, benefits may disappear. However, MSM can also contribute to the healing process and after some point may not be needed any longer. In any case, MSM can be taken for a long period of time.

Q: *Will taking MSM interfere with my medication?*

A: MSM has great potential as a nutritional supplement that can be used to support medical treatments. After many years of clinical use, it has not been found to interfere with any prescribed medication.

It is worth repeating that the healing effects of MSM often allow cutting back on prescriptions and sometimes even eliminating medication. However, never make the decision on your own. If you are under medical care, inform your physician first about your intention to take MSM. Show this book to your physician. Only your doctor should advise you whether to cut back or not.

MSM and blood tests: We have done numerous blood chemistry workups on patients and found that MSM does not cause any abnormal readings—with one exception. If you are scheduled to have liver function testing and are taking MSM, you should stop the supplement for about four days before the test. MSM has never been found to cause liver damage but it may interfere with the accuracy of the test for liver enzymes by sometimes producing false positives. Elevated enzymes are an indication of a liver disorder. You can resume the supplement after your liver test.

Q: *Are there any interactions between MSM and other medications?*
A: DMSO has been found in studies to counteract platelet aggregation. MSM has not been similarly tested in scientific studies for this effect, but clinical observations indicate it may have a blood-thinning, aspirinlike effect on platelet aggregation as well.

Platelets are structures found in the blood that play a major role in clotting. Excessive platelet clumping can form dangerous clots that participate in narrowing of the arteries associated with heart attacks and stroke.

Aspirin has been known for about twenty-five years to help reduce clotting activity, and millions of people take it as a cardiovascular preventive agent for this reason.

Our concern is that anyone taking high doses of aspirin, or blood-thinning medication such as heparin or dicumarol, should exercise caution when using MSM.

It is not known if MSM can play a beneficial role in preventing cardiovascular disease. This potential deserves to be investigated, given the interest in cardiovascular research to find effective anticoagulant agents.

However, if MSM is taken along with proven blood-thinning agents, an accelerated blood-thinning effect cannot be ruled out. Indications of such an effect might be the development of bruises on the body or increased bleeding from hemorrhoids.

If you are taking blood thinners such as heparin, dicumarol, or aspirin on a regular basis, we strongly recommend you consult first with your physician before using MSM as a nutritional supplement. If your physician approves, start at a low dose of MSM, perhaps one gram a day, and then very slowly increase dosage to an optimum level. Be certain to have your coagulation parameters monitored frequently. If any signs of bleeding appear, check immediately with your physician.

Q: *Is it safe for a pregnant woman to take MSM?*

A: Clinical experience indicates that MSM is safe for pregnant women. We recommend, however, that you consult first with your physician before taking this or any other supplement or medication.

Q: *Can a child take MSM?*

A: Children usually don't need MSM as a nutritional supplement. Parents whose children have allergies, asthma, or an inflammatory illness such as juvenile rheumatoid arthritis should refer to the chapters on those conditions and consider the use of MSM as an addition to regular treatment.

Many children have taken MSM, some in very large amounts, without any problem.

Q: *What if my child or my dog swallows a lot of MSM?*

A: MSM is very safe. If you determine that a child has swallowed this or any other supplement or a medication, the child should be evaluated by your physician or at a hospital emergency room. If your pet has swallowed a large amount of MSM, the animal could possibly develop diarrhea. The reaction would depend on the amount ingested. If you have any doubts, take the animal to your veterinarian.

Q: *I'm allergic to sulfites. Does that mean I will be allergic to MSM?*

A: Don't confuse MSM with sulfites. MSM is a sulfur compound but it is not a sulfite. The body produces sulfites in its normal metabolism of sulfur-containing amino acids. Sulfite compounds have been used for more than three hundred years and are generally considered safe. Currently they are used to control microbial growth and prevent browning and spoilage. However, an estimated half-million people are sulfite-sensitive in the U.S. Most often they are asthmatic adults and predominantly women. Reactions in non-asthmatics are very rare. Most reactions are mild and include a constricting of the bronchial tubes (the main reaction), GI symptoms, and behavioral changes.

According to the Feingold Association of the U.S., negative publicity prompted restaurant owners and supermarket managers to discontinue the practice of treating foods in salad bars with sulfites. However, they are still used for other foods, in particular grapes, wine, potatoes, and dried fruits.

If you have a sensitivity to any sulfur-based preservative, here are the names to watch out for:

- sulfur dioxide
- sodium sulfite
- sodium bisulfite
- sodium metabisulfite
- potassium bisulfite
- potassium metabisulfite

Q: *What is the best way to mix MSM crystals in liquid?*

A: Many patients like to take MSM crystals dissolved in liquid. This is particularly useful if you take higher doses and don't want to swallow a lot of capsules. Over the years, people have said that the "MSM cocktail" is the most effective way of taking higher doses.

Simply dissolve the crystals in distilled, spring, or regular water. MSM dissolves better if the water is heated to some degree. You can even take it in coffee and tea. The heat will not affect the MSM. You can also use juice or any other drink that is palatable and agreeable with you.

You may want to avoid milk. Many people are allergic to it.

Soda pop isn't a favorite choice of ours because of the excess sugar and other unhealthy ingredients. However, if a child refuses the MSM in water or juice, then soda may be your only option.

The No. 1 choice is simple water.

The maximum amount of crystals you can dissolve in room-temperature water is the equivalent of about 15 percent, or one-sixth, of the total volume of the liquid. If the MSM content is higher, the crystals will not entirely dissolve and the liquid may appear somewhat cloudy. However, there is no problem drinking the mixture even if the crystals are not entirely dissolved.

You can dissolve a higher percentage of MSM crystals if the liquid is warmer.

A 15 percent solution would be the equivalent of putting slightly less than a level teaspoon (just under five grams) of crystals into one ounce of liquid.

Q: *How do I use MSM topically?*

A: Repeatedly throughout this book we have recommended the parallel use of topical preparations as an additional vehicle for bringing MSM's healing properties into the body. We believe that MSM can be more beneficial when used in combination, that is, taken orally as a nutritional supplement as well as applied to the skin.

A variety of lotions, creams, and gels are on the market. Our preference is for a product as pure as possible. Our experience with topical formulas is primarily related to gels containing only MSM blended into a standard gel compound.

We are aware that some topical products contain MSM plus other ingredients. We have no information whether these other ingredients will enhance results.

We recently heard an interesting comment from an Arizona man regarding topical MSM. He said he had been using a commercial MSM lotion for a stubborn facial skin condition but wasn't having significant results. He decided to fortify the lotion with crystals from the MSM supplement he was taking. He found that if he first ground the crystals into a fine powder in a coffee grinder that the powder dissolved more readily into the lotion. He said the additional MSM made an immediate difference and cleared up a chronic dry, flaky, red rash in the area of his nose and cheeks. His successful formula was one-third powder to two-thirds of the lotion.

Q: *Is MSM available intravenously?*

A: We believe that the most effective way to deliver MSM in higher and more therapeutically potent levels to the body for very severe cases will likely be through the medium of intravenous infusions. Currently, this method is not generally available.

Many years ago when antibiotics where first used, they were given orally. In current practice, the intravenous method is employed for more complicated and critical situations.

MSM as an IV agent should be seriously investigated because the substance has the potential to provide substantial pharmacologic effects for numerous conditions for which we presently have no effective treatments.

Chapter Four

MSM and Pain

Relief for Four Damaged Bodies

Case #1: A Vietnam War Injury

Thirty years ago Corporal Mel Shiota of the U.S. First Cavalry Division jumped out of a helicopter into a Vietnam battle zone with forty-five pounds of machinegun, ammunition, and other equipment on his back. As he landed, he wrenched his left knee, the same knee, as luck would have it, that he injured playing high school baseball.

"I saw stars and could barely walk, but in a situation like that you just grit your teeth and keep moving," recalls Shiota, now fifty-two.

Twenty years later, the pain came alive again in his bad knee, the probable result of degenerative arthritis from the long-ago injury and the constant squatting and kneeling he does in his work. Shiota operates an automotive body shop in Los Angeles. He is continually up and down.

"My knee has been getting progressively worse," says Shiota. "In the morning, it would be so stiff and painful that I would have to manipulate the joints for a few minutes in bed before I could get up. At work, I would moan and groan every time I had to squat. I began having to take two or three Tylenol a day over the last four or five years."

Then Shiota heard about MSM from a friend and started taking half a teaspoon of crystals twice a day.

"It took about three or four weeks and I noticed I could get out of bed in the morning without so much pain and stiffness," he says. "It's been about six months now and more than half the pain and stiffness are gone. I don't need the Tylenol anymore."

(Case #2:) A Korean War Injury

Nick Puccio's wartime legacy of pain dates back more than forty-five years to the Korean War. The sixty-eight-year-old retired U.S. Army Signal Corps lieutenant colonel developed a painful trick knee stringing telephone lines in rugged mountain terrain and also returned home with "jungle rot" of the feet. Every summer for decades he would develop painful, cracked, and bleeding skin between his toes.

"I had been suffering for a lot of years until I started using MSM gel both on my knee and my feet," says Puccio, who lives in Fairfax Station, Virginia.

"The pain in my knee was frequently pretty intense and would interfere with my walking. Whenever I took a misstep it would get worse. X-rays never showed anything wrong. I refused to use pain pills and just lived with the pain. Now I massage some MSM gel into the knee whenever it flares up. The pain starts easing up within twenty-four hours."

Puccio first started using the gel around 1990. He says it "cured" the painful bleeding between the toes of both feet.

"This was a very miserable condition," he says. "Every summer, whenever it was hot, this condition would come back. My socks would become bloody. I tried every skin medication available and nothing worked. I was pretty amazed at what the MSM did. I used the gel for three months and the next year it didn't come back."

Case #3: Carpal Tunnel plus Accident-Related Arthritis

J. Tomita, forty, of Agoura Hills, California, has it all: carpal tunnel syndrome, a repetitive strain injury from working as a grocery cashier years ago, along with bad arthritic pain in the back, knees, and hips stemming from a 1984 automobile crash that nearly killed her.

"The pain has been so bad sometimes that I couldn't sleep. Practically every major bone in my body was broken, so you toss and turn all night because you can't get comfortable," says Tomita. "I don't like to take pain pills but I was taking Vicodin on a regular basis just to survive."

Tomita is a wife, mother of a four-year-old, part-time actress on TV soap operas, and manages a jazz band.

On bad days, she says, she would limp through her real-life and TV roles because of the pain.

"I can't limp when I'm filming though. The script doesn't call for it. So if the pain got bad enough, I would just swallow my pain pills to get through the work."

That was before MSM.

Tomita is amazed at the relief that came within two weeks.

"I can be totally productive again without a problem. I take a teaspoon of crystals three times a day and that generally keeps the pain down so I can handle business, the household, and my four-year-old girl. I sleep at night now and I really feel much more rested. If the volume of the pain goes up, I just take more MSM to bring it down. If I forget to take the MSM for one day, the pain soon lets me know. In my back. In my hips. In my knee. In my wrists. I'm not curing anything. Just managing the pain and inflammation without any pain pills. But that's all I need with my banged-up body."

Case #4: A Living Hell for Twenty-Five Years

At an age when most people are looking up the road ahead toward approaching retirement, Kaye Kolkmann was studying for her master's degree. She earned it in 1992 at the age of fifty-three. Now she's teaching English, and loving it, at two northern California community colleges.

What makes her accomplishment even more impressive is that she hurdled her way over the obstacle course of higher education carrying a heavy load of pain on her back. Starting at the age of six she was involved in a series of automobile accidents that progressively battered nerves, muscles, and bones in her neck and back. The cumulative injuries and inflammation created a narrowing of the spinal column surrounding the main thoroughfare of nerves running up and down the body—the spinal cord. The constriction produced excruciating pain.

"It was a living hell for twenty-five years," says Kolkmann. "There have been many times when the pain was so unbearable that I would just walk and pray the whole night through."

In the beginning, doctors prescribed barbiturates and other painkillers. But the pills tore up her stomach and spaced her out to the point where she couldn't effectively handle the responsibilities of raising three children. Besides creating new problems the pills only helped minimally with the pain. She took them for a while and then stopped.

Her best source of relief has been MSM, she says.

"I've gotten some relief from aspirin, but the MSM is what took the big edge off the pain and enabled me to carry on and accomplish my goals. There have been times when I couldn't concentrate because the pain was so bad. MSM reduced the pain enough so that I could work, study and otherwise function. It also increased my energy level. The pain is still there. It never goes away. But the MSM makes it bearable. I take it up to three or four times a day whenever the pain gets oppressive."

About Pain

Pain comes in many shapes. As pain specialist Ben E. Benjamin, Ph.D., noted in his book *Listen to Your Pain* (Penguin), it "can be mildly annoying or excruciating. It can be sharply piercing, it can be a dull ache, or it can tingle or burn. The cause of your pain might be a torn ligament or tendon, a pinched or bruised nerve, a broken or diseased bone, or even an emotional or psychological problem."

Basically, pain is an electrochemical SOS, your body's way of telling you that something is wrong. As one British medical expert dryly put it: "It is a warning of tissue damage and its persistent nature has a protective function by ensuring that the subject cannot ignore it except with considerable voluntary effort."

The message of pain starts with nerve endings at the location of damage on or in your body. The impulse travels from there at warpspeed along nerve fibers to your brain. The message says you have a dull ache here, a sudden fracture there, or a *screaming* headache. The brain then integrates your past and present experience and computes the significance of the pain along with an appropriate response.

To understand better how this works, and how MSM benefits you, let's take an example of somebody who burns a finger while cooking.

In a flash, the pain signal zips from your finger along a speedway of nerve fibers called alpha-delta fibers. These are fibers encased in fatty, protective tissue—myelin sheaths—designed for lightening-fast delivery of pain information to and from the brain. Alpha-delta fibers are part of the nervous system's sensory apparatus, which also includes alpha-beta fibers that conduct the sensations of touch.

In a millisecond, the message slams into your brain. "Ouch, it's the tip of the index finger on my left hand."

"Get your finger out of there," the brain shoots back in another millisecond. You instantaneously move your hand away, through the activation of another nervous system network, the motor system, that commands your bones and muscles.

There's a third network called the autonomic system. It controls such things as blood flow, blood vessel dilation, flushing, and perspiration. After the burn, the area of your fingertip starts to become red, and you feel a generalized pain in the end of the finger. This is the action of the so-called small non-myelinated nerve fibers (C fibers), which are part of the autonomic system.

The non-myelinated fibers are now taking over, conducting general messages of pain following the establishment of a "circuit," so to speak, between the brain, and the damaged area.

The alpha-delta fibers are more involved in the business of immediate, protective, and acute pain. The small non-myelinated fibers are more involved in the business of after-the-event and chronic pain, such as the kind associated with arthritis.

This is a simplification of a highly sophisticated and complex system, but it gives you a picture of a basic concept.

Both fiber systems extend from the peripheries of your body, in this case from your finger, up the arm, across the shoulder, and then connecting to your brain.

Both systems carry impulses—along different nerveways—up to the thalamus in the base of your brain, a walnut-sized switchboard that receives and relays warning signals and pain messages. From there, impulses are forwarded up into the brain. Specifically, they go to the cerebral cortex that registers the location and extent of damage, and to the limbic region atop the brainstem that deals with emotion. If the pain impulses are intense enough, the alarm bells sounded in the corridors of the limbic system will set in motion such responses as crying or sadness. It is precisely because of the limbic system that pain is now conventionally treated not just with painkillers but with drugs that deal with the emotional component of pain such as anxiety, fear, and depression.

Painkilling drugs—analgesics—range from over-the-counter aspirin to heavy-duty narcotics. They work by stopping the nervous system's normal functioning in some way. These pills perform the humane mission of eliminating pain while hopefully a healing process is taking place. The problem is that these drugs, in order to be strong enough to do the job, are often counterproductive to healing. They create toxicity in the body, interfere with normal metabolic activities, and create harmful side effects that add new problems to existing ones. This is particularly true if they are used regularly over a long period of time. In the case of narcotic analgesics, for instance, the body builds up a tolerance for and a dependence on the drugs. Higher and higher doses may become necessary to be effective, which may lead to lifetime addiction.

One type of painkilling medication—the nonsteroidal anti-inflammatory drugs or NSAIDs for short—are among the most commonly used drugs in the world when inflammation accompanies the pain problem. For more on anti-inflammatories, see the next chapter on inflammation. These drugs are notorious for their side effects.

MSM and Pain

At the DMSO Clinic at Oregon Health Sciences University, MSM has been used in the treatment of many patients with a variety of painful conditions. The supplement has proven to give significant pain relief in a majority of cases, perhaps 70 percent. Among the remainder, it has had only minor effects or none at all. There is, of course, no substance, whether a drug or a natural remedy, that works in every case. MSM is no exception.

The following is a list of some of the many conditions for which we have personally observed pain improvement with the use of MSM:

- severe accident-related pain
- degenerative arthritis
- rheumatoid arthritis
- fibromyalgia
- back pain from herniated discs, arthritis, and other causes
- headaches
- muscle soreness

- tendinitis
- bursitis
- carpal tunnel syndrome
- interstitial cystitis
- scleroderma
- athletic strains and sprains
- cold sores
- shingles
- TMJ
- Bell's palsy
- Buerger's disease
- inflammatory bowel disorders

We have also heard from many people we have not personally treated who have said that MSM provided relief.

As noted earlier, MSM has many of the actions of DMSO. Research has shown that DMSO inhibits the transmission of pain impulses along the C fiber network of nerves, producing a fast and stable analgesic effect. It is along this pathway that deep, aching pain is conducted. Such pain is involved in arthritis and musculoskeletal injuries.

In a 1993 study conducted at Southern Illinois University, researchers concluded that conduction of pain impulses is slowed down even with low concentrations of DMSO. Many years before, an experiment demonstrated that DMSO blocked C fiber pain impulses within a few moments. To date, no studies have been conducted to test this effect with MSM. But, our clinical observation over many years makes it clear that MSM is a strong analgesic.

To our knowledge, there have never been any DMSO or MSM studies done on the alpha-delta fibers, which conduct the impulses of sharp, first pain. So we do not know if there is any impact at this level.

However, other studies on DMSO have shown that it can produce a temporary blockage of central pain response in the brain. That's where pain is perceived.

One researcher years ago concluded that DMSO produces an analgesic (painkilling) effect by acting both locally and systemically, that is, on the level of C fibers and in the brain. The researcher compared this effect to morphine.

Keep in mind that DMSO is a prescriptive agent. Worldwide it is used extensively for trauma and many painful conditions. In the U.S., it is approved as a therapeutic agent for interstitial cystitis. By comparison, MSM is a nutritional supplement. On its own it has very substantial pain-reduction powers, even though it may not be quite on a par with DMSO.

Our clinical observations indicate that MSM possesses a number of the same pain-relieving qualities of DMSO, such as:

- An anti-inflammatory action (see the next chapter).

- An ability to soften scar tissue (see the section on scar tissue in Appendix A).

- An ability to dilate blood vessels and enhance blood supply. This suggests a supportive role in speeding the arrival of nutrients involved in tissue repair to damage sites in the body.

- An ability to reduce muscle spasm. Many pain conditions, whether disease or trauma related, have an accompanying muscle spasm component.

- The potential for rendering cell membranes more permeable. This may facilitate a greater effectiveness of the body's own natural painkillers.

In one respect MSM has a major advantage over DMSO. As mentioned earlier, MSM does not generate the fishy breath or body odor as does DMSO. This nuisance factor often discourages people from continuing with DMSO on a long-term basis even though it is doing them a world of good. If you are looking for long-term relief of pain and don't want to be annoyed by an odor, MSM is the natural solution.

Unlike pain pills and anti-inflammatory drugs, MSM does not

produce any serious side effects. If you take too much for your individual constitution, you may have some temporary gastrointestinal reaction, such as increased frequency of stool. If you encounter this, reduce the amount you are taking. Keep in mind that each individual has a different level of tolerance.

As word about MSM spreads, patients are getting ahead of their physicians and trying the supplement on their own. Physicians frequently call us to ask about MSM after their patients tell the doctors how MSM has helped. One such doctor is David Blyweiss, M.D., of the Institute of Advanced Medicine in Lauderhill, Florida.

"This is patient-driven," Blyweiss told us. "Patients come to me and say that their pain is 50 percent better or more on MSM. A dozen people have told me that. None of them has mentioned any negative effect."

Among the patients who have reported improvements to Blyweiss are individuals with rheumatoid arthritis, scleroderma, polymyalgia rheumatica, fibromyositis, and other pain and connective tissue disorders.

"The patients tell me they start to feel better within a week," Blyweiss added. "They talk of having less fatigue, better sleep, and better ability to exercise. All these effects are downstream from having less pain."

In Wheeling, Illinois, chiropractor Richard Schaefer, D.C., says that he first heard about MSM from a medical doctor whose patients were taking it and reporting relief from pain.

"I have now been recommending MSM for more than six months," says Schaefer, who treats mostly musculoskeletal conditions. "The results have been excellent. I consistently see major reduction of pain and inflammation in the area of arthritic joints, along with improved range of motion. MSM is effective for your typical wear-and-tear arthritis, post-traumatic injuries, low back and neck pain, muscular pain, and tendinitis. Patients experience relief within five days to two weeks on average and I can't think of a single individual who isn't getting some kind of a positive effect."

Accelerated Healing

Some of the physicians who contact us for information on MSM are nutritionally oriented practitioners. They include medical doctors, osteopaths, chiropractors, and naturopaths. These are health professionals who employ many different nutritional supplements in their healing protocols. They often tell us that when they add MSM to an already existing program for a patient they see accelerated healing and marked improvements, often in cases that have been resistant to other treatments.

One physician, for instance, mentioned this accelerating repair effect of MSM for a number of his most difficult patients who had degenerative and rheumatoid arthritis and other musculoskeletal problems.

"With MSM, patients show accelerated signs of repair, such as reduced pain, increased range of motion and neurologic coordination, and joints returning to more normal shapes and positions," he commented.

Such accelerated healing for a resistant condition was recently reported by one of our patients, Richard Liss, 45, of Malibu. Liss, a professional masseuse for twenty years, had developed a chronic muscle strain just below his right shoulder blade as a result of the repeated forceful movements that his work required.

Liss had been taking high doses of Motrin on an almost daily basis for nearly a year. He was also seeing an acupuncturist for the pain, taking a full range of vitamin supplements, receiving deep tissue massages on his back, and regularly applying cold packs to the affected area.

Despite all his efforts, Liss says he was not getting significant relief for his pain.

"The pain had taken over and become the focus of my life," he says. "It would often wake me up in the middle of the night. It would be there when I awoke in the morning. It would be there when I worked on clients. I am not in a position to stop working, so I had to adjust my technique and rely more on my left arm and less on my right arm and just push through the pain. I had to stop playing tennis because that had become too painful. The whole thing was a nightmare."

Liss started taking 3 grams (3,000 milligrams) of MSM in late spring of 1998. Three months later the pain level was about 20 percent of what it had been before.

"I haven't needed a Motrin in two months," Liss says. "Within one month it was clear that the MSM was accelerating my healing. The pain had dramatically subsided and reached a nondebilitating level. I could get on with my life. I am not 100 percent, and I may never be 100 percent again as long as I continue to do massage work, but the pain is no longer on my mind very much, and no longer ruining my life. I am also back to playing tennis, and I couldn't do that before MSM."

Over the years, many people have have told us that MSM has accelerated their recoveries following surgical procedures.

Recently, Carol Davis, 64, a housewife from Indian Shores, Florida, told us her surgeons were surprised at the speed of her recovery following knee replacement in mid-1998.

"I had been taking MSM for about three years," says Davis, who has a history of painful joints and muscles from years of skiing, playing racket sports, and involvement in other recreational activities. "The MSM has enabled me to deal with the pain in the past because I am not one to take medication. I know that it really helped me because if I missed taking it for a few days the pain would become worse.

"Even though the pain was tolerable with the MSM my right knee had deteriorated to the point where much of the cartilage was gone. Walking became impossible. I had to get around for a while on crutches and a wheelchair. My doctors first tried an arthroscopic procedure in February of 1998 but that didn't work. That's when they said I would need a full replacement. They offered a strong analgesic prescription but I refused. The MSM was giving me enough relief as long as I didn't walk.

"In June I had the knee replaced. I kept taking a very high dose of MSM before and after surgery—a total of about 40 grams daily in divided doses. The hospital provided me a morphine pain pump but I hardly used it. The nurses were surprised.

"Afterward, when I went to see my orthopedic surgeon for a three-week checkup, he said that the status of my recovery was more like three months. He was very surprised."

At three months, Davis says she is "doing great. I'm not dancing yet, but I may soon. I'm walking slowly and have a solid 90 degree flex of my knee."

Questions That People Ask Us about MSM and Pain Relief

Q: *How does MSM kill pain?*

A: We believe that MSM relieves pain in at least several ways:

1. It inhibits pain impulses along a major nervous system network called C fibers. These fibers carry messages of pain from a site of damaged tissue in the body to your brain.

2. MSM also reduces inflammation. Inflammation puts pressure on nerves and other tissues and causes pain.

3. MSM promotes blood flow, which enhances the healing process.

4. MSM reduces muscle spasm—a contraction of muscle tissue—often involved in painful conditions.

Q: *Will MSM help with both acute pain that comes on suddenly or develops after a traumatic event, as well as chronic pain related to arthritis or some other disease?*

A: Usually it helps in both circumstances. Almost always, acute pain responds more rapidly than long-standing chronic pain. If you incur a sprained ankle or fracture, MSM will probably help reduce the inflammation and you may have some pain relief as a result. If you have suffered from a pain-related disease for many years, you need to be patient and give MSM time to get into the system and work.

Q: *I have heard people who have been in pain for a long time say they have had dramatic overnight relief.*

A: This does happen. We have personally seen cases where people experience great relief within a few days. Such dramatic responses are not unusual and are very gratifying to both physicians and patients. However, we advise patients who have been suffering from chronic pain for many years not to expect overnight relief. Although it is very possible to happen sooner, the first signs of relief could take one month, two months, or even many months to become apparent. If you are not among the fortunate individuals who experience relief in the days or weeks after you start taking MSM, don't be discouraged. Stick with it. Be patient. You may not notice less pain immediately, but you may feel more energetic from the MSM, or you may experience other side benefits (see Appendix A on the additional benefits of MSM).

Q: *How long does it usually take to experience relief in very severe cases?*

A: This is difficult to answer. It depends on many things. Some severe cases can take months. The longer the problem has existed, the longer it may take for substantial relief to occur. Often MSM helps where nothing else does, where there are no other effective treatments available, or where strong medication is not advisable for a patient. The use of MSM may provide major relief or it may provide just enough to allow your physician to reduce the amount of medication. When a doctor can do that, the risk of side effects is also reduced.

Q: *Is pain relief from MS lasting or temporary?*

A: That's another hard question to answer. It depends. Many people experience relief as long as they keep taking the MSM. When they stop, symptoms return. There are a number of case histories in the book that describe this. Sometimes the symptoms will return quickly if you stop the MSM. Sometimes they may take weeks or months or even years to return. Or they may never return. MSM speeds the healing process. Once the body is healed from an accident, the pain may vanish only to return again at a later time in the form of degenerative arthritis that often follows in the wake of trauma. Continued use of MSM might help retard the onset of arthritis-related pain in such cases. We have observed a number of cases where patients have had remissions from serious illnesses, such as lupus and interstitial cystitis. They have taken MSM on a regular, long-term basis and this has probably contributed to their recoveries. If you are obtaining relief from pain associated with chronic illnesses, you will generally continue to experience such relief as long as you take the supplement.

Q: *If I develop pain should I take MSM?*

A: MSM can be helpful for many cases of pain, but remember that pain is a messenger from the body telling you that something is wrong and needs attention.

A minor pain that comes and quickly goes is generally not a cause for concern. But when any pain intensifies or persists, that's a strong message you should heed. As pain expert Ben E. Benjamin, Ph.D., notes: "There are many people who fail to listen to their body's early warning signals, and as a result they have compounded their injuries, crippling themselves with unnecessary pain for months and even years."

Be alert to minor pain whenever it occurs. Consider any repetitive activity you do as a possible cause of pain. If you take action right away you can prevent minor aches from developing into chronic severe pain problems later.

Persistent pain can ruin your life. It can affect your ability to learn and concentrate, to perform routine daily tasks, or to care for your family. In the worst cases, persistent pain can lead to anxiety, a dependence on medication, drug-induced side effects, additional health problems, and even a tendency to commit suicide.

Should you experience any kind of severe or persistent pain, for whatever reason, don't rush to the health food store and buy a bottle of MSM and expect it to relieve your pain like a painkiller. MSM doesn't work that way. It is not a pharmaceutical pain pill that will deaden the pain in ten minutes. See your physician. Get a diagnosis and follow your physician's advice.

If you have a stabbing toothache, see a dentist. MSM may help cut the pain but you need to address the cause of the pain.

If you develop acute appendicitis, don't rely on MSM for immediate relief. See a physician immediately.

If you have a splitting acute headache, don't start taking MSM capsules and expect them to work like Advil.

MSM provides rapid relief in many cases, but it is not meant to compete with pharmaceutical painkilling drugs. It is a nutritional supplement. MSM is most appropriate for chronic pain conditions where you don't want to rely indefinitely on a drug. If you have a chronic pain condition, MSM can be used along with any therapeutic program you follow. It will not interfere with any drug or procedure being administered by your health professional.

Q: *How much MSM should I take for pain relief?*

A: For severe pain you may need to take at least two heaping teaspoons of crystals (each level teaspoon is five grams) a day.

Dosage is very important. The general rule is to take as little as possible but as much as you need to obtain the desired level of pain relief. Each of us have individual needs. A level that works for one person may be too little or too much for a second person with the very same condition.

To give you an idea of how you can find your individually effective dose, consider the example of Cheryl Brown, who manages one of our medical offices (Lawrence's). Brown, 46, started taking MSM in the spring of 1998. She has three medical problems: 1) osteoarthritis in the neck with bone spurs, a degenerative condition that developed after two automobile accidents some years before, 2) migraines that occur once or twice a month, and 3) discomfort and slight pain in the wrists, the beginnings of a carpal tunnel–like condition related to computer overuse. She took several medications for the control of the arthritis and migraine pain but was experiencing minor stomach upset and was not happy about having to continue the drugs on a long-term basis.

Brown began taking two 750-milligram capsules of MSM a day, one in the morning and one in the evening after work. Within two weeks, she noticed the pain in her wrists disappeared, even when she put in long days at the computer.

She then doubled the dosage, to the equivalent of 3 grams (3,000 milligrams) daily. "I got pretty good pain relief with that, but it wasn't quite good enough," she says. "Some of our patients were coming in and describing phenomenal relief. I wanted the same thing for myself."

Brown then increased the MSM to 4.5 grams (4,500 milligrams) daily, her current level. "The increase made a huge difference," she says. "It seemed to be the dosage my body needed. My head felt clearer. The arthritis pain almost vanished. The range of motion in my neck improved. I was able to rotate my head much further toward my shoulders than before. I feel I am now in good shape again like when I was younger."

Brown says she has not needed to use any pain medication—with the exception of an aspirin a few times—since raising her MSM level to 3 grams.

Jeffrey Marrongelle, D.C., a nutritionally oriented chiropractor in Schuylkill Haven, Pennsylvania, uses MSM for patients with headaches, muscle pain, and arthritis. He finds that initial improvement is usually followed by slow, steady progress.

"By then raising the dosage substantially, according to individual patient tolerance, we can often achieve additional benefits more rapidly," he says.

It makes no difference whether you take capsules or crystals. If you need to take more than just a few capsules a day, you may find that crystals are more convenient. You should note though that MSM has a bitter taste. Some people don't mind the taste; others do. You can add the crystals to water, juice, or any other liquid. They dissolve more readily in warm or hot water, so you can even add them to tea or coffee.

Always start with a lesser amount and then work up slowly to the individual dosage that provides maximum pain relief. If you take too much MSM at once, you may encounter some gastrointestinal discomfort. Reduce the level or take the MSM in divided doses during the day to prevent such discomfort.

If you are under the care of a physician, tell your doctor what you are doing. You may find you are able to reduce your pain medication by taking an MSM supplement.

Q: *Besides taking the MSM orally, what else can I do to help my pain?*

A: Apply MSM topically in the form of a gel, cream, or lotion, which are available commercially. MSM has the ability to pass through tissue. It will pass through the skin and enter into your system. This additional dose of MSM increases the pain reduction and healing effect. Apply the MSM topical product to an affected area of your body to generate a local anti-inflammatory benefit. Refer back to Chapter 3 for more information about MSM gels, creams, and lotions.

Q: *If I take MSM, should I stop the prescription I am using for pain relief?*

A: MSM may provide substantial pain relief in many cases but do not stop taking your regular medication until you consult with the health professional who is caring for you.

Chapter Five

MSM and Inflammation

They Said She Wouldn't Walk Again:
Beverly Spencer's Story

Inflammation follows trauma like night follows day. In Beverly Spencer's case, she developed massive inflammation following a 1986 automobile accident.

Spencer, of Lake Oswego, Oregon, was riding in a car that had come to a complete halt at a stop sign. Suddenly, it was rammed from the rear by a car traveling nearly seventy miles per hour. The driver had been under the influence of cocaine. The impact crushed several discs in Spencer's back and neck. She was totally bedridden for eight months.

"The doctors told me I would never walk or work again and the best I could look forward to was going on outings with other handicapped people," she says.

"After the accident, I had very little movement in any part of my body," she relates. "There were parts of my body that were black and bluish-gray from the bruises and lack of circulation. I hurt so much any time I tried to even slightly move. But I knew I had to try, even with the pain. I have raised four children and worked all my life and it wasn't like me to lie in bed. I spent all of my time figuring out how I was going to get out of bed and get well again."

The medical reports were not encouraging and her doctors didn't give her any hope of functioning normally again. She had major post-traumatic inflammation and muscle spasm in the back and neck. She took painkillers and a muscle relaxant every few hours to help her through the ordeal.

"In 1987, after months of being bedridden, I learned about MSM and started taking a teaspoon in orange juice twice a day," she says. "It took a few weeks before I felt anything. First I started gaining some circulation. The color of my skin improved. There was growing feeling in areas that had been numb. I started slowly gaining movement. First in my hands and arms. I noticed there was less pain and I didn't have to use the pain pills as much. Eventually I was able to stop them altogether. There hadn't been much improvement until I started on the MSM. But now I felt I was slowly getting better.

"After three or four weeks on the MSM I found I was able to start rolling over and actually get out of bed and go to the bathroom myself. Even though the bathroom was six feet away it took me two hours to go and come back.

"I had horrendous pain, when I was lying in bed or if I got up. The MSM helped to alleviate the pain. I would take a dose at noon and by four or five in the afternoon I would have quite a lot of pain again. Then I would take more MSM and within two or three minutes I would feel better. Gradually the intensity of the pain decreased. After four months on the MSM I could slowly walk to the living room and actually sit up for a few minutes at a time."

Spencer says it took her a year and a half before she could walk comfortably or do simple household chores. Her doctors were amazed that she could even do that much. After she became ambulatory, she walked with a pained, almost palsied gait that caused people to turn their heads or look away.

"I would have to throw my legs out to the side and bring them around in a circular movement in front of me to get them moving," she remembers.

Spencer made an amazing recovery. It took her three years of working through pain and slowly building up atrophied muscles. Today, at age fifty-seven, she is her usual "workaholic self," as she admits, logging 100-hour weeks as owner and operator of a Montessori school. Recently, she and a friend laid 3,800 bricks in the school patio and installed new playground equipment at the school. She routinely moves tables and cabinets on her own.

Although her ordeal is behind her, Spencer still has to be careful.

"I am pretty strong for such an injured woman but I can't bend down and pick things up," she says. "I have to squat and take objects in my arms and then stand up. My discs are crushed and if I make the wrong move I go back to bed. I have had a few relapses.

"I don't have any pain now to speak of. If I do, I just take an extra dose of MSM. I don't know where I would be if it hadn't been for the MSM."

Spencer isn't cured by any means. The severe injuries she incurred inevitably led to degenerative arthritis in the neck and back. The MSM won't reverse the arthritis but it helps relieve the associated pain.

MSM offers powerful relief for individuals with inflammation, whether it stems from an inflammatory disease process or, like Beverly Spencer, from trauma.

MSM and Inflammation

Inflammation is a complex reaction of the body whenever its cells or tissues are damaged through disease or injury. You can develop chronic inflammation over time in the degenerated joints of osteoarthritis or in the muscles and joints associated with rheumatoid conditions or as the result of injury. You can also develop acute inflammation due to burns, radiation, venom, or infections.

Inflammation is associated with a number of characteristic signs that have been described since the ancient Greeks and which all medical students learn early on in their education. They are:

- rubor (redness)
- calor (heat)
- dolor (pain)
- tumor (swelling)
- loss of function of a particular body part(s)

MSM is a bonafide anti-inflammatory agent and impacts each of these inflammatory signs wherever present in the body. In hundreds of cases, we have seen swelling in patients go down, felt localized heat normalize, and observed the redness decrease and become more like the normal color of skin. Patients themselves attest to the pain reduction and normalization of function.

One of the primary properties of DMSO is its ability to render the body's own natural anti-inflammatory hormone more effective at lower doses. That hormone is cortisol, produced in the adrenal glands. Cortisone, also known as steroid medication, is the pharmaceutical version of our own cortisol. In a laboratory study conducted many years ago, researchers found that the presence of DMSO stabilized—that is, helped protect—vulnerable cellular components against a variety of damaging agents even when cortisol concentrations were ten- to a thousand-fold less than normal. This means that it takes considerably less of the body's own natural anti-inflammatory agent to protect cells when DMSO has been introduced.

MSM may also have this medically important action. Over the years, and for many inflammatory conditions, the use of MSM has permitted a reduction in the dosage of cortisone necessary to control the swelling. We have seen this effect repeatedly in cases of rheumatoid arthritis, among the most inflammatory of disease processes known to medicine.

Another shared inflammatory property may be the inhibition of fibroblastic proliferation. Fibroblasts are the primary cells of the body that form connective tissue. They transform into different specialized cells that make up the fibrous, supporting, and binding tissue of the body. Excess fibroblasts are produced in the swelling process and eventually lead to scar tissue. DMSO reduces fibroblasts and also binds to fluids in swollen tissue and takes them out of the body.

Muscle spasm often accompanies inflammation. MSM also has a muscle-relaxing effect that reduces spasm.

A Caution on Anti-inflammatory Drugs

For many years, the medical community has recognized the problem of adverse drug reactions, particularly in the stomach and intestinal tract, caused by nonsteroidal anti-inflammatory drugs that are used by tens of millions of patients for the relief of pain and inflammatory conditions. "The most prevalent serious drug toxicity in the United States is increasingly recognized as gastrointestinal pathology associated" with these drugs, an article in a 1991 issue of the *American Journal of Medicine* stated.

At a forum on pain in July 1997 conducted by the American Medical Association in New York, patients were warned about ulcers and other medical problems that arise from prolonged use of widely prescribed and over-the-counter anti-inflammatory drugs.

"It's a public health problem," said Michael B. Kimmey, M.D., a gastroenterologist at the University of Washington Medical Center in Seattle.

Data cited at the forum from the "Arthritis, Rheumatism and Aging Medical Information System" indicate that approximately 76,000 hospitalizations occur each year in the U.S. from gastrointestinal complications produced by nonsteroidal anti-inflammatory drugs (NSAIDs). An estimated 41,000 hospital admissions and 3,300 deaths involving elderly patients are attributed annually to NSAIDs.

Fifty to 80 percent of people admitted to hospitals with gastrointestinal bleeding are taking NSAIDs, according to Kimmey. "Every time they come in with bleeding, they have a 10 percent chance of dying," he says. "I don't think people realize that until it may be too late."

The most common side effects are stomach pain, indigestion, ulcers, hemorrhage, and perforation, which can lead to death. Kidney damage is another frequent consequence of regular use of NSAIDs.

In many countries, non-aspirin NSAIDs are the most frequently used drugs. Such usage increases with age, primarily for osteoarthritis and other chronic musculoskeletal problems. Studies have shown that on any given day 10 to 20 percent of elderly patients are taking an NSAID prescription.

Aspirin is the most familiar NSAID. But more powerful NSAIDs include compounds with ibuprofen, naproxen sodium, and ketoprofen. Such products are available in both prescription and over-the-counter form.

A key problem, according to Kimmey, is that many over-the-counter NSAIDs are taken by people without a good reason, which puts them "at risk for a catastrophic problem. Most of these drugs are not taken because doctors advise people to take them. People see advertisements and they go and get them without talking to a doctor."

A Canadian study in 1996 warned that NSAIDs should be avoided if possible, particularly among the elderly and other high-risk patients. "Currently, no NSAID is available that lacks potential for serious toxicity," the researchers said. Another Canadian study indicated that many physicians were overprescribing NSAIDs for the elderly.

At a 1998 San Diego conference of leading orthopedic surgeons attended by one of us (Lawrence), the issue of NSAID side effects was a frequent topic of conversation. Most experts there believed that these medications should never be used for longer than five or six days.

Steroidal anti-inflammatories are commonly prescribed by physicians when the nonsteroidal versions of medication don't work. Steroid drugs, including cortisone, are really wonder drugs as long as they are used for short periods of time and in very small doses. That is how most doctors use them. When necessary and when used properly, steroids can save lives and rescue people in crisis, such as in cases of acute asthma or allergic attacks. Usually, when taken for a week or less, they are safe. Some patients, in fact, actually feel stronger on steroids.

The problem with steroids is when you take them for a longer period of time. That's when you run the real risk of serious side effects. And that's a dilemma often faced by people with rheumatoid arthritis or certain neurological disorders suffering from agonizing pain not brought under control by milder medication. As bad as the NSAID side effects may be, the consequences of prolonged cortisone use are much worse.

Common adverse patient reactions include gastrointestinal irritation and bleeding, suppression of the immune system and increased susceptibility to infections, retention of fluids and a swollen appearance, broken blood vessels and black-and-blue marks, weakness, interference with sugar metabolism, and a tendency to develop delusional behavior. Many people fear steroids because of the side effects and for good reason.

On Friday, August 7, 1998, the major networks announced the arrival of a new drug—called Arava—for the treatment of rheumatoid arthritis, the most inflammatory arthritis condition. The drug had earned the unanimous endorsement of an FDA advisory panel. Such recommendations are usually followed by the government's approval of a drug for medical sale and patient use.

Newspapers around the country carried the details the next day. *The Los Angeles Times,* for instance, ran an Associated Press report about the drug under the headline "A Breakthrough for Victims of Arthritis." The report said the following:

● Arava is the first in a series of "promising new treatments approaching the market" in more than a decade for rheumatoid arthritis.

● It does not cure rheumatoid arthritis but appears to work as well as the "gold-standard treatment"—the cancer drug methotrexate—which is known to cause "troublesome side effects" and whose effectiveness diminishes over time.

● The manufacturer, Hoechst Marion Roussel, conducted a year-long trial with 480 patients with moderate disease. Of those,

41 percent experienced improvement compared to 19 percent who said they improved taking dummy placebo pills.

- X-ray studies of bone erosion and cartilage disappearance were conducted to determine the progress of the disease. Arava patients "did get worse," the article said, but placebo patients "worsened four times more quickly."

- Arava caused side effects, including diarrhea and hair loss, in more than a quarter of all patients. "But Arava did not seem as prone to causing the serious problems that methotrexate sometimes can, such as kidney failure," AP said, quoting one of the doctors who monitored the study's safety.

- But the drug has a "significant problem," the article continued. Most drugs dissipate quickly after the last dose is taken. Arava can take at least six months to clear.

- "Also," AP said, "animal studies suggest it can cause numerous birth defects." The advisors warned that pregnant women should not take Arava and that pre-menopausal women should guard against becoming pregnant if they use the drug. "More troublesome was what to tell women who have already taken Arava and then decide they want to have a baby," the report continued.

- Finally, the advisors recommended regular liver monitoring, "because just like methotrexate, Arava can cause liver damage."

We have no comment on this "promising" new drug. The article says it all.

By comparison, there are no serious side effects associated with MSM. You can take it for virtually every condition where an anti-inflammatory drug is prescribed, including rheumatoid arthritis (see Chapter 20). If you develop inflammation as a result of trauma, burns, or any disease process, MSM can be a highly beneficial add-on to treatment. Take it orally. Apply it also topically as a gel or lotion to any area of inflammation on your body.

Oral MSM helps relieve inflammatory bowel conditions such as Crohn's disease and ulcerative colitis. Crohn's usually affects the lower segment of the small intestine, causing both severe pain and diarrhea. The diarrhea, in turn, leads to painful irritation and inflammation in the perineal area between the anus and the genitals. MSM helps reduce the inflammation in the gut, which will lessen pain and diarrhea. This in turn reduces inflammation of the perineal tissue.

Ulcerative colitis involves inflammation of the inner lining of the colon and rectum. The effect of MSM here is the same as it is with Crohn's. Patients report a lessening of symptoms and a more normal stool size, color, and frequency. Ulcerative colitis is associated with an increased risk of colon cancer.

Both of these conditions often generate secondary inflammation in the joints. MSM helps reduce the inflammation in the joints as well as the intestines.

Part **TWO**

How **MSM**

Helps Relieve

Common Pain

Problems

Chapter Six

Arthritis (Osteoarthritis)

"I will see you back for surgery": Ellen Nelson's Story

Ellen Nelson delivers the mail in Littleton, Colorado. She carries a pouch that weighs upward of thirty-five pounds, for five and sometimes six days a week. She was doing just fine until she noticed her right knee starting to ache and stiffen up during the busy Christmas postal season of 1997.

Nelson shrugged it off as a reaction to the extra-heavy load of Yuletide parcels and cards as well as overtime. But in the month following the holidays, the stiffness increased and the ache turned into outright pain. She went to see her general practitioner. The doctor examined the forty-five-year-old mail carrier's right knee and concluded she had developed degenerative arthritis. Moreover, the doctor said, her other knee, even though it wasn't hurting at the time, appeared to be in even worse shape. The physician referred her to an orthopedic specialist who confirmed the diagnosis after additional X-rays and tests.

"The orthopedist prescribed physical therapy, knee braces, and 600 milligrams of ibuprofen daily," Nelson says. "As I left his office he said, 'I am pretty sure I will have to see you back for surgery on both knees.' "

Nelson began taking the medication and wearing the braces, which was difficult as her job involved a lot of climbing in and out of her mail truck.

"The condition worsened, and my left knee soon began hurting me worse than the right," she says. "The pain and stiffness were bad in the morning when I got up. I had to stand by the edge of the bed and move my feet up and down just so I could begin to function. If I stepped in a hole or stubbed my toes against a sprinkler head during my route, the pain would jolt my legs like electricity. Once or twice a week, the pain would wake me up at night, with my knees and shins involved. Sometimes I would also have painful night cramps in my legs as well. The pain medication helped take the edge off for a few hours but when it wore off the pain and stiffness would return."

Nelson, who had never taken prescription medication before, was uncomfortable with the prospect of long-term pain pills. Her physician wanted her to come back in six months for bloodwork to check for any possible adverse effects in the body from the medication.

"The thought of side effects, of damage to my liver or kidneys, was very disturbing," says Nelson. "I liked less the prospect of surgery."

Pain had suddenly entered—and upended—her life. She even had to stop going to movies because the pain didn't allow her to sit through a film.

In spring of 1998, Nelson struck up a conversation with a resident along her mail route who works as a salesman for a leading nutritional supplement company. During their chat, health issues came up and Nelson mentioned her problem with arthritis. The salesman then told her about how he had used a nutritional supplement to relieve a painful shoulder condition. He offered her a sample of the supplement and suggested she try it for a month. The supplement was MSM.

"I am basically a skeptic and I wouldn't have gone to a health food store to buy it," she says. "But I figured I had nothing to lose."

Nelson started taking three one-gram (1,000 milligram) capsules of MSM a day and continued with her pain medication. For almost a month she felt no difference. Then she began noticing improvement—less stiffness and pain in her knees.

"The improvement continued, and soon I had the same spring back in my legs just like I had before all this started," she says. "I was feeling major relief."

As her pain level dropped, Nelson weaned herself off the medication. Within two months, she discontinued it totally.

"I was pain-free," she says. "No pain in the knees. No cramps. I'm walking my route faster. One weekend I went for a long car ride, attended a baseball game, and climbed on my roof to trim some crab apple trees. I could never have done that before. I'm back to seeing movies. I feel like a new woman."

About Osteoarthritis

Wear and tear of the joints of the body leads to osteoarthritis, or, as it is called medically, degenerative joint disease. This, the most common form of arthritis, causes much misery as we get older and leads to musculoskeletal pain, the No. 1 chronic pain condition, according to the American Geriatrics Society.

Over time, the joints begin to degenerate from usage. Depending on genetic predisposition, your lifestyle, biochemical and hormonal changes, and what you do for a profession, the degeneration occurs earlier or later, faster or slower.

The facing bone surfaces in a joint are coated with a layer of cushioning tissue called cartilage. This soft and spongy material enables us to enjoy locomotion and movement in a painless manner. The cartilage ensures a smooth ride, a frictionless movement of parts, but it becomes damaged from years of wear and tear. This degradation triggers the production of enzymes that further damage the tissue. The result is gradual degeneration of the cartilage. It becomes rough, brittle, dry, and pitted. Inflammation occurs and can affect the synovial membrane (the tissue lining the joints) as well as adjacent tendons or ligaments. You experience stiffness, muscle strain, fatigue, decreased function of the joint, and pain. You have arthritis. Weight-bearing joints under the most stress are the most common trouble spots. They includes flexible bones in the spine, the knees, and hips. The shoulder, hands, and feet are also frequently affected.

According to the The Arthritis Foundation, 21 million Americans are affected with degenerative arthritis, mostly individuals over the age of forty-five. It is the number-one cause of disability for people over sixty-five—surpassing back pain, cancer, diabetes, and heart and lung conditions. After we turn the corner into the new millennium, the numbers are expected to rise precipitously as the growing wave of baby boomers hit fifty and sixty.

Conventional medical treatment focuses on a dangerous pharmaceutical barrage of painkillers aimed at silencing the pain associated with arthritis. From aspirin and acetaminophen, to cortisone and nonsteroidal anti-inflammatory drugs, these medications are neither corrective nor preventive. They, in fact, can be detrimental to the health of the patient if taken for a length of time.

NSAIDs, as we discussed in earlier chapters, are used widely for arthritis. However, these drugs are risky both to the patient and the patient's joints. NSAIDs work by blocking the action of enzymes that help produce inflammatory compounds. At the same time, however, the drugs also inhibit enzymes that produce components of cartilage. Thus, you may see some pain relief from NSAIDs for as long as you take them, but beneath the surface they may be actually accelerating the arthritic process!

Three Clinical Perspectives on MSM and Osteoarthritis

Perspective #1—Stanley Jacob, M.D.

MSM impacts osteoarthritis in the following ways:

- It reduces pain.
- It reduces inflammation.

- It reduces muscle spasm around arthritic joints, which also helps relieve pain.
- It lessens the formation of scar tissue.
- It improves blood flow throughout the body, including painful joints.
- It may slow down the degeneration of cartilage.
- It delivers biologically active sulfur to the body.

A number of medical studies over the years have indicated that sulfur levels in arthritic joints are lower than normal. In a 1995 study, sulfur concentration in arthritic cartilage was shown to be about one-third the level of normal cartilage. This figure was comparable to earlier sulfur measurements reported in *The Journal of Bone and Joint Surgery* and the *Journal of the Southern Medical Association* during the 1930s, which described the use of intravenous and intramuscular injections of sulfur for arthritis. These studies found the cystine content of fingernails to be 25 percent lower in arthritics. Cystine is a sulfur amino acid that helps build hard tissue such as fingernails and hair. In one of these older studies, when a group of 100 arthritics was given a solution of sulfur intravenously, pain was relieved in many cases and the cystine fingernail test returned to normal.

MSM offers major benefits for osteoarthritis. At this time we don't know precisely how the sulfur in MSM is utilized by the body to help arthritis, and whether, for instance, it directly contributes to the maintenance or repair of cartilage and joints. Sulfur-containing compounds called glycosaminoglycans are abundant in the cartilage and synovial fluid of joints.

In my clinic I have used MSM routinely for many years, often for severe, debilitating osteoarthritic cases where patients have traveled long distances seeking help. These are not minimal cases of pain and discomfort. MSM supplementation has provided significant improvement—less pain, less stiffness, greater mobility.

Some years ago I conducted a clinical experiment to compare the effect of MSM and NSAIDs. In the study, twelve female arthritic patients were randomly assigned to take a moderate dosage of 600 milligrams of Motrin three times daily. Motrin is a popular NSAID. Another twelve women were assigned to take 6 grams (6,000 milligrams) of MSM daily. After one month, the patients from both groups reported an approximately equal degree of improvement in terms of reduced pain and inflammation. Among the Motrin group, three patients complained of moderate discomfort from hyperacidity. Gastrointestinal complaints are common among NSAID users. No side effects were reported among the patients who took MSM.

This small clinical study, while not a rigorously controlled experiment, nevertheless demonstrates there are safe, effective nonpharmaceutical remedies for arthritis.

Many of my patients ask me about glucosamine sulfate, another sulfur compound enjoying current popularity as a remedy for osteoarthritis. Glucosamine is an organic component of connective tissue and cartilage. As a supplement it is said to help relieve symptoms and stimulate new cartilage formation.

A number of my patients have compared MSM to glucosamine sulfate. They have expressed the opinion that while glucosamine has given them varying degrees of relief, they feel that MSM provides even greater relief. Glucosamine sulfate is certainly worthwhile. In my experience, MSM is more effective for severe cases.

In 1997, one patient told me that she had better results when she took both MSM and glucosamine sulfate. There was less pain when she took both, she said, than when she took one or the other. I decided to test her observation and recommended to about two dozen osteoarthritis patients then taking MSM that they now add 1,500 milligrams of glucosamine, the generally recommended daily dosage. The feedback was quite positive. Less pain, the patients said. Thus there may be a synergistic effect from combining these two supplements.

As a tribute to MSM's potency, some supplement companies have already begun adding MSM to their glucosamine sulfate formulations.

Patients have frequently asked my opinion about chondroitin sulfate, another popular nutritional supplement suggested for arthritis. I have not seen patients improve after adding chon-droitin sulfate, however.

MSM often allows patients on medication to reduce the num-ber of pain pills they need and sometimes even eliminate them. If you are on medication, always consult your physician first before modifying or stopping a prescription. Some individuals have been taking cortisone for many years for its anti-inflammatory effect. In such cases, it is not advisable to stop taking it without medical supervision. You may not be able to eliminate the cortisone alto-gether. This is because once you take cortisone for a long period of time, your body's natural ability to produce its own cortisone—the anti-inflammatory hormone, cortisol—becomes diminished and may even be permanently suppressed. But MSM may allow you to reduce the dosage. But for your own safety, do not reduce this or any other prescriptive medication on your own, no matter how well you are feeling.

In some very severe cases, MSM has postponed the need for hip or knee replacement. An example of this was a 70-year-old patient with severe arthritis in both knees. His physician had rec-ommended double replacements, which in his case was inevitable. He was in pain when he sat and developed more pain when he walked even a short distance. He started MSM orally and topically and within two months began to walk with much less pain and stiffness. He felt a great improvement in his overall quality of life. If MSM can postpone surgery by even a year or two, as in his case, replacement techniques will improve and the potential for a more successful outcome will be enhanced.

Perspective #2—Ronald Lawrence, M.D.

The first of my pain patients to start on MSM was an 80-year-old woman with generalized arthritis. Her condition involved the fin-gers, hands, knees, neck, and low back. Like some of my other arthritic patients, she had been taking glucosamine sulfate for a year or more. With glucosamine, her pain had lessened by about

30 percent. After starting MSM, she reported an additional—and significant—reduction in pain.

As I began recommending MSM to my other arthritic patients, they would tell me the same thing. Within two to four weeks, sometimes sooner, they would start feeling better. Less stiffness. Much less pain.

One such patient was a 75-year-old lawyer who already had undergone two knee replacements. He also suffered from severe arthritis in both shoulders, feet, and the low back. I introduced him to MSM as an addition to an existing treatment program that included acupuncture. In about four weeks he reported feeling significant improvement in overall pain. As this book is being written, he has been taking three heaping teaspoons of MSM daily for seven months. He says his pain relief is substantial, and he also reports being more limber.

Tom Rodriquez, my gardener, had developed painful degenerative arthritis in his lower back and knees, the physical toll of nearly forty years of hard landscape work in the Los Angeles area.

"It is getting harder and harder to move around," he told me. "My legs feel heavy and just don't have the same power as when I was younger. You get older and you got to expect these things."

Tom, who is 69, said that at the end of a long work day, he was increasingly relying on aspirin or Tylenol to ease his pain. I gave him a supply of MSM and suggested he try three 750-milligram capsules daily. A month later, Tom told me that his pain was virtually gone.

"The pills you gave me helped plenty," he said. "There is just slight pain in the knees, but the back pain is gone. My legs are much more flexible and not as heavy as they felt before. I haven't taken aspirin once. I am very happy and I am not going to stop taking the MSM."

This kind of positive feedback from patients and friends prompted me to conduct a small clinical study to measure the pain-reducing power of MSM. Pain is a very subjective matter. Only the person suffering really knows how much he or she is hurting. It is hard to express the degree of pain verbally. For the purposes of this trial, patients were asked to assess their pain on a scale of 0 to 100 (100 being the worst pain) at the start of the experiment, again at four weeks after starting MSM, and again at six weeks.

In the study, subsequently reported in the *International Journal of Anti-Aging Medicine,* I took sixteen patients, aged 55 to 78, and randomly assigned them to two groups. One group of ten patients was given 2,250 milligrams of MSM daily. That's the equivalent of taking a standard 750 milligram capsule three times a day. The other six patients took a specially prepared placebo pill that matched the MSM in appearance and taste.

The experiment was conducted according to a "blind" model. This means that neither the patients nor I, as the overseeing physician, knew who were taking MSM or who were taking the placebo until the trial was completed. Records were kept by an independent evaluator.

The participating patients all had degenerative joint disease, confirmed by X-rays, and had suffered from severe pain for many months or years. They represented a cross section of arthritis, ranging from one joint involvement to a generalized condition. Most had used NSAIDs or aspirin-type medications for relief. None had taken steroids previously. All drugs or other nutritional supplements were stopped prior to the study.

All patients in the study reported improvement while taking MSM, except for one. At the four-week mark, patients on MSM described an average 60 percent improvement; at six weeks, 82 percent. As is typical in medical studies, people on placebos usually report benefits. In this case, the placebo takers described an improvement of 20 percent on average at four weeks and an 18 percent improvement at six weeks.

In this study, and in my general clinical experience, I find that many patients taking MSM notice substantial relief of pain within three to four weeks although some have reported major relief within days. As a result, I have often been able to reduce the dosage and sometimes even eliminate the use of strong hydrocodone painkillers, such as Vicodin.

The similar results of this limited trial, and that of Stanley Jacob in his Portland clinic, and another clinical trial by a Brazil-

ian doctor you will read about in a moment, invites a more inten-
sive investigation of MSM for the relief of pain related to degenerative arthritis. Such a broader study should involve a larger group
of arthritic patients and take into consideration additional evalua-
tions such as range of motion.

I have been treating pain for forty-five years and started the
first in-patient pain clinic in the country—in 1970—under the
auspices of the UCLA School of Medicine. I am keenly aware of
the limitations of standard pain medication. The side effects can
be devastating, worse even than the condition that the drugs are
supposed to treat. We physicians need to be extremely prudent in
prescribing them. For this reason, I am very excited when a natural agent such as MSM becomes available, can provide significant
pain relief without side effects, and enables me to lower the dosage
of medication. I find that it can be used along with any other prescriptive medication. To date, I have not seen any adverse interactions.

What has been very poignant to me as a pain specialist is the
experience of having dozens of osteoarthritis patients call me, or
drop by my office, after they start on MSM, and tell me how good
they are feeling, how much better their range of motion is, and
how they have been able to become more active in life. These are
people who have been suffering for years.

As impressive as the painkilling effect of MSM is on degenerative arthritis, in my experience it appears to be even more potent
for rheumatoid arthritis (see the section on rheumatoid arthritis in
Chapter 20). Some very severe, chronic cases have responded dramatically. Patients are surprised at how fast MSM relieves the pain
and inflammation. Some rheumatoid patients have told me they
started feeling relief within days.

Prior to using MSM, many of my degenerative arthritic
patients took glucosamine sulfate. I found it to be a helpful,
steady agent in about 35 percent of milder to moderate cases,
but it did not appear to be as effective in patients with severe
arthritis. MSM, in my experience, appears to be a more potent
agent in the most difficult patients and in general offers more
relief to more people. In addition, it has many side benefits that

glucosamine does not have. I haven't observed the same surprising and dramatic results with glucosamine usage that I have with MSM.

As I began recommending MSM, I didn't tell my patients already taking glucosamine sulfate to stop that particular supplement. I just suggested they add MSM. Generally, after about two to four weeks they would report a noticeable improvement in their condition. These were people who had been on glucosamine for six months or a year and had appeared to reach a plateau of benefit. Their additional relief was clearly due to the effects of MSM.

I have found that glucosamine usually takes four to five weeks before it kicks in. The fastest appreciable response by any of my patients with glucosamine was about three weeks. This is with the standard dosage of 500 milligrams three times a day. I haven't seen any improved results by increasing the dosage. MSM, on the other hand, appears to have increased benefits when you step up the amount you take. MSM, in some cases, can generate relief in a few days, but for severe, long-standing cases you need to give it time. In my clinical experience, such patience pays off.

Arthritis in the hip joint can be a serious problem. I haven't found glucosamine effective with severe joint disease in this location. Results with MSM are far superior. In severe cases involving the knees, I have found glucosamine only mildly effective—far less than 35 percent of the time among my patients. Again, MSM has been much more beneficial here.

I have found that glucosamine sulfate taken with meals produces no effect. It needs to be taken on an empty stomach.

We are now starting to see MSM being added to glucosamine products. It may be that a combination of the both offers some synergistic value and may be more beneficial. By the way, as far as cost is concerned, in the stores that I have checked, I have found that MSM is less expensive than glucosamine sulfate.

In my experience, chondroitin sulfate, another nutritional supplement said to promote healthy cartilage, has not proven to offer any significant clinical benefits. Scientific research indicates that chondroitin is generally not well absorbed.

Perspective # 3—Ephrain Olszewer, M.D.

In Brazil, Efrain Olszewer, M.D., director of the International Preventive Medicine Clinic in São Paulo, has been testing MSM on arthritic patients for more than a year.

"We wanted to see if arthritics could be maintained on MSM alone, without any medication such as nonsteroidal anti-inflammatories," says Olszewer. "The results to date are good in 90 percent of the cases."

Involved in the Brazilian physician's clinical study were sixty men and women, ages 40 to 82, with mild to moderate arthritis of the knees, hips, hands, shoulders, or spine. They were prescribed 750 milligrams of MSM twice daily. If one joint only was affected, Olszewer had them also apply an MSM lotion made especially for him by a local pharmacy.

His assessment of MSM: "We measure the mechanical movement of the involved joints and ask the patients about their pain and stiffness. We have measured greater motion and flexibility in the joints. The patients have told us they have much less pain and stiffness. Patients say the pain relief starts usually within the first fourteen days. In a few cases, as early as within two days. We haven't seen any kind of side effects or intolerances of the patients. In a few patients it didn't work at all."

Two Painful Arizona Knees

Doug Ohmart operates a health-food store in Tucson and says he has tried every supplement on the market to help relieve the chronic pain in his left knee. The arthritic pain is a legacy from his high school gymnastic days when he severely injured the knee.

"My doctor says the cartilage is like mush," says Ohmart, 44. "It's really bad degenerative arthritis in the joint. I have just suffered through the pain, which is always there. Whenever it gets intolerable, which is maybe twice a month, I will take an ibuprofen prescription. At times like that I can just barely walk on it."

When glucosamine became popular a few years ago, Ohmart started taking the supplement but says it didn't help much.

"It didn't do anything to speak of for the pain or the flexion," he says. "I took it for eight months."

In 1997, he first heard about MSM and started taking it—a half teaspoon twice a day in his regular protein drink.

"I couldn't believe what happened. In two days, there was a huge reduction in pain. Huge. It was like a gift from heaven. I don't know if it was the MSM and glucosamine working together. I have no idea. I only know that right after I started the MSM there was this major improvement.

"What's more, I have regained a lot of the lost flexion in my knee. As a result of my injury and arthritic condition I only had about half or less of the normal flexion. Before MSM, if I laid on my back and brought my knee up to my chest and then pulled down on the ankle, I couldn't get it within two feet of my rear end. Now I'm only about ten inches away. I've regained a lot of bend, although for me the prospect of being able to bend the knee so I can sit back on my heel is a pipe dream. As far as pain is concerned, it's not entirely gone, but my worst day now with pain is like my best day before MSM. I haven't had to take any ibuprofen since MSM."

Early in 1998, an enthusiastic Ohmart related his experience to Gary Sebring, a security guard at a Tucson electric utility company, whose job requires walking regular rounds of two six-story buildings. Arthritic pain in his right knee was making the job torture.

Says Sebring: "Because of the pain I would often limp along, take the steps real slow and use the railings for support, and when anybody was around I would just pretend I was fine. I had considered getting a cane but a security guard with a cane doesn't project the right image. I was concerned I might need a knee replacement."

The knee pain had started a year before and increased over time. "At the end of the workday I would just come home, sit down in pain, and hardly be able to get up," he says. "That wasn't like me. I like to go fishing and camping but I could hardly even stand in the boat to fish anymore or barely climb forty feet without taking a rest. I stopped all my outdoor activities because of the pain. I couldn't walk from my front yard to the back without some pain."

Sebring says he tried glucosamine sulfate for a month but had no relief. Then Ohmart told him about MSM. "After hearing his story I decided to try it as well, so I started taking about a quarter or half a teaspoon twice a day," says Sebring. "Within three or four days, the pain practically disappeared. It was pretty amazing. It's been about eight months and now there is only slight pain when I overdo it. I handle the walking routine at my job now without any problem and even go on three-mile walks a few times a week for exercise. I couldn't do that before. I'm also back to fishing and camping and have no trouble walking up and down the banks of streams. It's great. My knee isn't like it was when I was sixteen but compared to before it feels like a new knee."

Sulfur Baths and MSM "Soaks"

From time immemorial, arthritis sufferers around the world have made healing pilgrimages to hot mineral springs, rich with the odoriferous but soothing properties of sulfur and other minerals. There they soak in, and drink down, the waters in an effort to ease their painful joints.

Can hot sulfur springs actually benefit arthritis? Definitely, says a scientific assessment of sulfur baths on arthritis that appeared in a 1966 issue of the German medical journal *Praxis*. In the report, researcher E. Maibach monitored 120 subjects with various degrees of arthritis. Most of the patients were between 50 and 60 years of age.

"After removing from consideration hopeless cases of degenerative arthritis of the spine (9 cases), the results after 10 baths showed improvement in 61 percent (68 patients), with 17 percent (12 patients) of this total being symptom free," the researcher concluded.

Maibach said that the criteria of improvement included subjective reports of less pain and increased mobility of stiffened joints, as well as X-ray evidence of affected joints. The participants in the study also drank the sulfur-rich water, suggesting that benefits may have occurred not only from through-the-skin penetration of sulfur and other minerals, but also from oral ingestion.

The Maibach study included a review of the medical literature and cited previous experiments indicating that concentrated sulfur extracted from mineral baths passes through the skin of both human and lower animals. This is consistent with clinical observations demonstrating that topical MSM, in the form of gels, lotions, or creams, passes through the skin and into the body. For this reason, we recommend the use of these topical products for additional local and general benefits.

Recently, a Canadian businessman who had been taking MSM orally for shoulder, back, and knee pain, set out to replicate the sulfur springs effect in his own home—he installed a special hot tub and added MSM crystals.

"I have gotten considerable relief from the supplement but the old healing tradition of mineral springs led me to think that if I soaked in MSM maybe I could get better results," he says. "I played a lot of hockey in my younger days and my joints got banged around pretty good. As a result I've been suffering a lot with degenerative arthritis. I hadn't been able to jog for about five or six years because of the pain. Now, after I finish hot tubbing, I can go out and jog. And according to my wife, the hot tubbing has put extra bounce in my stride. For me, the greatest benefit of tubbing has been increased flexibility and decreased stiffness, particularly in my lower back, but all my joints have benefited from the soaks. I now soak myself in MSM every day."

His personal experience with MSM suggests a possible use of "MSM soaks" for athletic training, physical therapy, and rehabilitation clinics (refer to Chapter 10 on muscle pain to see how one athletic coach is using "MSM soaks").

MSM and Heberden's Nodes

Heberden's nodes are arthritic bumps on the finger joints. Take MSM orally for this condition, but also apply MSM gel once or twice a day to the affected joints. It will take considerable time, probably many months or even a year, but your patience may be rewarded with a reduction in the pain and size of the nodes.

If you don't have any gel available, soak your fingers in a luke-warm—but not hot—solution of MSM. Use about 15 percent MSM in the water, that is, one part MSM crystals dissolved in six parts of water. Do this for at least a half hour at a time, perhaps while watching television. To maintain the temperature of the water, you can use an electric foot bath device available at most pharmacies.

"The Energy Side Effect"

Many people who take MSM say they feel more energy. From Fritz Meyer, of Castle Rock, Colorado, comes the suggestion that older folks who take MSM for arthritic joints should be careful of the energy boost it delivers.

Meyer introduced his mother, Mildred, to MSM around Thanksgiving of 1997. Mildred is 93. She had painful and stiff knees, and experienced difficulty rising from a chair and discomfort when walking.

"Within six weeks or so she was greatly improved, taking three of those 750-milligram capsules a day," says Meyer. "She couldn't believe how good her knees felt. She could walk practically pain free and get up from the chair without complaining.

"But she also got this great infusion of energy. She felt so good she thought she could take on the world and so one day she felt so energetic that she got down on her hands and knees to wash the floor of her kitchen. She hadn't done that in a long time, a very long time.

"At that age you don't have the cushions and flexibility you have when you are younger. She pulled ligaments, damaged her knees, and put herself out of commission for a long while. She keeps taking the MSM, which we believe is helping her mend, but it was a real setback."

The lesson in this story is that even if your joints are improved and your battery becomes recharged, take it easy. Go slow. Don't overdo it.

Down in Tucson, Lou Salyer, 77, also experienced the energy buzz of MSM after she started MSM for painful arthritic knees and hips. She also admits to overdoing it afterward, but unlike Mildred she didn't damage herself in the process.

In her words: "For a long while I have had the blahs. I had no stamina. I had to force myself to get things done around the house. After two days on that MSM stuff it was like a blast of energy. I went out and did all the weeding that I had been putting off. At the end of the day I was exhausted. I did more than I should have. But my husband had had a stroke and there was so much weeding to be done in the yard. I just felt so good I decided to go out and finish the job.

"The amazing thing is that the next day my energy was right back up again and it's been up ever since. I take my half teaspoon of powder every day, and I am amazed at how much I get done now. This has been going on for a year."

As for the reason she took MSM in the first place, Salyer says her joints hardly hurt anymore.

Chapter Seven

Back Pain

A Hairdresser's Relief:
Liz Miners' Story

For more than three decades, hairdresser Liz Miners has been standing on her feet for many hours five days a week cutting, styling, coloring, straightening, and waving the hair of her clients—and listening to their problems. Eventually she developed a serious problem of her own—back pain.

Miners, 55, owns and operates Lizanne's Hairdressing Salon in Burlington, Ontario, southwest of Toronto. Five years ago she had to start reducing her work day because of the increasing pain.

"Two doctors told me I had degenerative arthritis from all the years of standing and I definitely had the pain to prove it," she says.

Miners says that her pain required her often to sit down between clients, "ooing and awing a bit," as she put it, and having clients wait until she could resume work.

"At the end of a long day, the pain would really bother me," she recalls. "In the morning, after a night's rest, it would be better but after standing for an hour or so in the salon it would start to get bad again. Work was becoming very difficult and I couldn't sit comfortably in the car when I drove home."

Miners tried an anti-inflammatory drug but quit after a few days when it gave her an upset stomach. Subsequently she went for regular physical therapy and chiropractic treatments that gave her some relief but not enough to more than take the edge off the pain. She still had to rest between clients to prevent the pain from becoming more severe.

In 1996, Miners heard about MSM and started taking one or two teaspoons a day.

"It gave me relief that no treatment or doctor had been able to give me," she says. "The pain began melting away within days and there was substantial relief within a week or ten days. In a couple of months, the pain was 85 percent gone."

Even with all her relief and comfort, Miners pampers herself and maintains a reduced schedule.

"I don't think my back will ever be 100 percent normal again," she says. "If I work six hours or so without a break then I can start to feel a little twinge in the back but nothing compared to what it was before. Compared to most people in my situation I think I am doing great. If I work less or take regular breaks, then I have no discomfort at all. But I wouldn't want to be without the MSM."

About Back Pain

If you have back pain, you are not alone. Seven million people are temporarily out of work at any given time due to low back pain and 80 percent of adults will eventually experience back pain at some point. According to the National Ambulatory Medical Care Survey from 1980 to 1990, back pain is the fifth most frequent reason for doctor visits (behind hypertension, pregnancy, check-ups, and upper-respiratory infections).

Even the super-famous are not immune—Elizabeth Taylor has suffered from recurring back pain for years.

For the famous and not-so-famous alike, chronic lower back

pain—and the leg pain that often accompanies it—adds up to the single most expensive health-care problem and the most common cause of disability for persons under the age of 45. The annual combined cost of back-pain related care and disability compensation is reaching $50 billion in the United States, according to Richard A. Deyo, M.D., a back-pain specialist at the University of Washington. This is truly a dynamic growth industry. The cost of back pain is up from $20 billion just a dozen years ago.

And don't think that only adults are affected. Half of American children develop low back pain by age 12!

What is interesting, in fact a "paradox," Deyo says, in a 1998 article on back pain in *Scientific American,* is that work disability has steadily risen despite an increasingly post-industrial economy with less heavy labor and more automation.

The causes of chronic back pain are many. They include:

- Arthritic changes in the spine, a result of wear and tear.

- Calcium deposits (spurs) develop as a result of spinal stress, trauma, nutritional and genetic factors, and especially wear and tear. They can dig into neighboring soft tissue and cause pain.

- Disc herniation (also known as a ruptured or slipped disc).

- Sprains of the ligaments that connect muscle to the backbone.

- Misalignments (called subluxations by chiropractors and lesions by osteopaths, who are experts in treating back pain) in the spinal joints or sacroiliac joint that connects the backbone to the hip bone. Misalignments can occur at any time in life, from spinal trauma during childbirth, bad posture, accidents, or sedentary lifestyle.

- Repetitive stress injuries (RSI) involve micro-trauma to the body's tissues that accumulate over the years, and are usually related to activity or jobs that people perform repeatedly. Repeated twisting, lifting, pulling, jogging or running, for instance, can cause back pain.

• In many cases, the psychological stresses that accumulate through daily life settle into the back, causing muscle spasms and pain.

Conventional treatment emphasizes painkillers, anti-inflammatories, and surgical solutions.

In recent years, we have seen studies in major medical journals revealing that a majority of people with spinal abnormalities, including protruding, herniated, and degenerated disks, do not have back pain. Often when such abnormalities are found through MRIs and other sophisticated imaging techniques, patients are referred for unnecessary surgeries.

Interestingly, Americans have almost ten times more spinal disk operations than people in other Western countries, according to a 1994 article in *The New York Times* that quoted John Froymeyer, M.D., of the University of Vermont. "Perhaps not coincidentally, there are also far more neurosurgeons and orthopedic surgeons in the United States, and many times more MRI machines," the *Times* said.

The findings of the MRIs are often misleading and lead to "unnecessary surgery and the results are not very good," Froymeyer said.

Another expert, Robert Boyd, M.D., an orthopedic surgeon at Massachusetts General Hospital in Boston, said, "Surgery doesn't put new backs in and it doesn't give better long-term results. It is indicated when pain doesn't respond to conservative treatment and is clearly associated with nerve root compression. Then the results of surgery are excellent." But only a small percentage of people with back pain fall into this category, according to Boyd.

In recent years, the treatment of low back pain with chiropractic manipulation has received powerful approval from government agencies in the U.S., Canada, and the United Kingdom. In Canada, for instance, the Ontario Ministry of Health's Manga Report of 1993 overwhelmingly endorsed the efficiency, safety, scientific validity, and cost-effectiveness of chiropractic for low back pain. A year later, the U.S. Government's Agency for Health

Care Policy and Research endorsed the use of spinal manipulation as a first line of treatment for low back pain.

Stanley Jacob, M.D., Comments:

I have seen too many patients who have had two or three back surgeries and suffer with more pain than they had before. I believe conservative treatment should be used whenever possible, unless there is so much pressure on the nerve that it is causing interference with basic functions in the body.

MSM has an important role to play in the nonsurgical treatment of chronic back pain and should be considered as a partner in any conservative approach, such as chiropractic and acupuncture. MSM won't diminish the size of a protruding disk or eliminate the basic problem; however, it relieves the inflammation around the disc. It is this inflammation that compresses and irritates the root nerve coming out of the spinal cord.

I have seen several hundred patients for back pain secondary to osteoarthritis, lumbar stenosis, disc degeneration, spinal misalignments, or accidents. For such pain-related conditions, MSM is usually beneficial. There may, in fact, be no pharmaceutical therapy that is better. Drugs, of course, can produce serious side effects.

In my experience, it generally takes a higher level than normal of MSM to relieve back pain (see Chapter 3 for dosage recommendations).

Ronald Lawrence, M.D., Comments:

I have found MSM extremely helpful for early gradations of back pain that include muscle strains, ligament sprains, and the early degenerative changes involving the vertebral joints and discs.

In my experience, I haven't found it as helpful in cases of advanced disc disease, but I believe it is worthwhile to take anyway as a supportive supplement. Keep in mind that MSM inhibits the transmission of pain impulses along nerve fibers, produces a reduction of inflammation, and reduces muscle spasms. Since inflammation, pain, and muscle spasms are all often involved in these situations, I believe MSM can provide some extra benefits and relief even for severe cases.

For these reasons I have made MSM a part of my therapeutic program for patients with herniated discs. My recommendations include gentle exercise, ultrasound, acupuncture, hot baths, massage, Tylenol, and, if needed, mild muscle relaxants.

Golfers often develop disc problems because of the powerful force they exert on their backs when they swing. I treated a lawyer, an avid golfer, who had developed intense pain in his lower back. An MRI showed that he had five millimeters of disc protrusion, a moderate herniation. He came to me because he wanted to avoid surgery and I suggested he give my multifaceted approach a chance. Within three months, his pain had diminished to an ache, and then it gradually disappeared.

Another patient had a disc that was out eight millimeters. He also went on this program. Six months later he was given another MRI and the protrusion had retracted to four millimeters. I feel that in cases such as these the MSM plays a useful therapeutic role and substantially supports the overall treatment.

Two More Cases of Relief

Case #1: Patience Pays Off

In 1968, during a long and difficult delivery of her first child, Hermine Zubko, then twenty-four years old, suffered a hairline crack of a spinal bone in her lower back.

"I felt a searing pain, as if a rod of lightning struck me," she recalls.

In the weeks and months that followed, Zubko experienced intermittent severe back pain. She resisted taking medication because, as she says, "I have a high tolerance for pain."

Over time, however, the pain became constant and frequently

disabled her. "There were many occasions when I couldn't sit, bend, stand, or walk without excruciating pain," she says. "Often I couldn't sleep because of the pain. Once, after watching a movie, I couldn't rise to my feet and had to be carried from the theater."

Zubko, who lives in Newberry Park, California, was forced to give up her hair salon business. The pain had become overwhelming, forcing her to try anti-inflammatories. She took them off and on for two years but "They gave me stomach pain and diarrhea. I didn't need more problems and one day I just threw them all out."

The minuscule fracture in her spine eluded detection by contemporary X-ray and other diagnostic methods for many years and Zubko suffered through her pain without knowing the cause. Two physicians told her flatly they thought the problem was all in her head. Another sent her home to perform a series of exercises, which did not help.

Later, through MRIs and more sophisticated medical diagnostics, Zubko was found to have severe arthritis, inflammation, and thick scar tissue at the site of the original trauma. Degenerative arthritis is frequently associated with back pain. In Zubko's case, the arthritis developed as a consequence of the injury to the spinal bone tissue as well as the aging process.

Following her diagnosis, an orthopedic surgeon initiated a treatment program of cortisone injections along with physical therapy three times a week. The program, however, was unsuccessful. The pain continued. Another specialist offered her "some glorified aspirin" but said basically there was nothing he could do for her.

By now, in the mid-1980s, she had been in pain for more than fifteen years. "I had practically lost all hope and wanted to die because I couldn't stand the constant pain anymore," Zubko says.

Zubko's salvation from pain came as a result of conversation during a physical therapy session. Her therapist mentioned that he had heard about people with severe pain being helped at the DMSO clinic in Portland. Zubko called and made an appointment in April 1984. Her condition suggested she could benefit from regular use of MSM.

"I started taking MSM crystals a few times a day in juice," she says. "First a quarter teaspoon, then a half, and then a full teaspoon. It took quite a while, but Dr. Jacob kept encouraging me to continue. He said it would take time. He said that for some people results come fast and for others it takes longer, that each individual and each condition is different."

For Zubko, it took eight months.

"One day early in January of 1985 I woke up and I was literally pain-free," she says. "There had been minor improvement to that point, yet the previous day there was still quite a bit of pain. In fact just before Christmas I had obtained another supply of crystals and I remember that I hadn't felt all that much better than when I started. It was really an overnight change. One day pain. The next day no pain. I couldn't believe it. Suddenly I could sit, I could walk, I could bend. It was like a miracle. I was able to work again full-time and regain my life."

Zubko had developed severe arthritis over a long period of time. In many cases, the longer a person has arthritis and the more severe it is, the longer it takes for MSM to produce results.

You might wonder how the pain could disappear from one day to the next after many months of taking the supplement. In her situation, there was likely a very gradual reduction of inflammation and pain until one day she passed a threshold where the pain level is reduced to the point where it is no longer perceived by the brain. Even though she still has degenerative arthritis of the back, Zubko has been able to enjoy a pain-free existence and function normally as long as she keeps taking the MSM.

(Case #2:) Heartburn Improved and Back Pain Gone

Paul Lisseck, 52, president of a marketing company in Amherst, Massachusetts, started taking MSM because a friend said it could help his esophageal reflux, a condition associated with heartburn. Lisseck had developed increasing discomfort, "a heaviness in the chest," as he put it, after eating. It was most apparent after spicy foods.

Lisseck began to notice some relief from the MSM shortly

after he started it but what really impressed him the most was the effect on his back pain.

"I injured myself in a fall years ago, and after I reached 45 I began to have pain in my lower back," says Lisseck. "According to doctors, the pain was probably due to a combination of the injury and wear-and-tear arthritis. Besides, I do a lot of driving in my work. Everything was just accumulating into back pain and it was giving me fits."

The pain developed to the point where Lisseck went for chiropractic treatment.

"The chiropractic helped. I had many sessions. But the pain kept coming back and I was hesitant to do anything requiring the use of the lower back," he says. "Amazingly, the MSM I was taking for the heartburn seemed to work wonders for my back. The back suddenly took a turn for the better and over the past three months I have not experienced any of the pain and tightness I normally have. I have been taking other supplements for years but when I added MSM that made the difference."

Chapter Seven

Headaches

About Headaches

Headaches are painful not just for the people who have them but for the doctors asked to treat them. In a 1994 survey conducted by *Consumer Reports* magazine, medical treatment for headaches was voted the single largest category of patient dissatisfaction—nearly 25 percent.

Such discontent implies a huge number of people. Nearly half of all Americans experience at least one headache a month and about 10 million of us (4 percent of the population) are moderately to severely disabled by different forms of headaches.

The vast majority of headaches are related to combinations of muscle spasm at the back of the neck and changes in blood vessels feeding into the head. Tension is frequently an underlying cause and can be generated from emotional stress, fatigue, misalignments of the cervical spine, premenstrual pain, nutritional deficiencies, eye disorders, and medication.

Experts say that many headaches and migraines are brought on by the very same medications intended to eliminate them, a phenomenon known as "analgesic rebound." It can be caused by aspirin, acetaminophen, ibuprofen, and other analgesic drugs when taken in excess. The effect is apparently similar to a drug dependency, where patients experience withdrawal symptoms and exacerbation of headache on abrupt cessation of analgesics. "Increasing demands for pain medication should arouse a suspicion of the development of rebound headaches," said a 1997 report in the medical journal *Hospital Medicine.*

If you take an aspirin or another analgesic medication, you often receive symptomatic relief quickly.

Don't think about MSM as an instant fix as you would a painkiller. It probably isn't going to give you relief in ten minutes—although some patients have said it does.

Here is what MSM can do—and can't do—for headaches:

- MSM usefulness is primarily for chronic headaches related to tension and muscle spasm.

- Migraines basically have a vascular causation. We haven't found that MSM reliably relieves migraine headaches. However, migraines may often involve a fair amount of muscle spasm and tension in the neck, which can contribute to the pain. MSM is worth trying for its ability to reduce muscle spasm.

- Taken regularly as a nutritional supplement, MSM inhibits certain pain impulses in the body as well as reduces inflammation. See the chapters on pain and inflammation for more details. MSM also appears to have some anti-tension properties, although we don't know the exact mechanism.

- Don't ignore the use of MSM topically as an additional avenue of relief. Apply MSM cream, gel, or lotion to the back of the neck where you feel tension. Do this frequently, perhaps every hour or two. MSM can reduce spasm of skeletal muscle tissue under the skin in the area where it is applied. Some of the MSM appears to act within the skin tissue to reduce surrounding tension, while some of it enters into the bloodstream and circulates in the body. Many whiplash patients have used MSM in this fashion—applying it to the skin, as well as taking it orally—to help obtain relief from headaches. Muscle spasm in the neck is associated with whiplash (see Sue Watson's story following the next one).

The following case histories show that MSM has the potential to offer relief from headaches stemming from widely different causes. Such cases, and observations we have made clinically, suggest that a person taking MSM orally or using it topically may often be able to lessen the intensity of chronic headaches.

"No more vises": Lynne Chauncey's Story

Lynne Chauncey, 57, a Portland housewife, is among the longest users of MSM. In 1978, she had been suffering for about a year from severe tension headaches, night sweats, and hot flashes, the menopausal after-effects of a hysterectomy.

"The headaches felt as if somebody was squeezing the top of my head in a vise," Chauncey remembers. "There was no pattern to them, except that they would always be there and the least little bit of emotional stress would make them worse. Even making a decision in a restaurant—did I want soup or salad?—could increase the pain. I took a lot of buffered aspirins but they didn't help much. I would often wake up in the middle of night bathed in sweat with my head pounding."

A friend of Chauncey's was a female patient who had just started taking MSM and had experienced some relief from gastrointestinal discomfort. The friend suggested she try the crystals and see if they could help her problem as well.

"I tried the crystals. What happened next I never dreamed would happen," says Chauncey. "The very first night I had no night sweats, no hot flashes, and no more pain. Perhaps I have a weird physiology but I never had another problem as long as I kept taking the crystals.

"My effective dose is a tablespoon of crystals every morning. I will take more, maybe a tablespoon three times a day, if I feel I am coming down with something or my allergies start to flare up. I used to have severe hayfever allergies, with sinusitis, sneezing, itching eyes, runny nose, and a hacking cough. I would have the problem every spring. In the fall I would have bad allergic reactions to mold. I still have problems with the itchy eyes now and then, but I don't have any infections or other heavy-duty symptoms.

"In the beginning there were times I would forget to take the MSM because I was feeling so good. I was soon reminded that I needed to keep taking the MSM because I would then start developing a hot flash or the viselike pressure in my temples. When I resumed the crystals the symptoms would disappear. So I just made MSM part of my daily routine and learned not to let my supply run out."

A Not-So-Merry Christmas Tale:
Sue Watson's Story

Christmas day, 1997, was not so merry for Sue Watson of Lake Oswego, Oregon. She was home nursing a painful headache, wearing a neck brace, and sore all over—the aftermath of a double whiplash injury. Two days before, while driving home from dropping off gifts to friends, she was rear-ended not once but twice in an automobile accident. Watson, a thirty-nine-year-old office administrator, was waiting for oncoming traffic to clear in order to make a left turn. At that moment she was struck from behind and then once again when a second car slammed into the vehicle that hit her. Watson's head was suddenly jolted backward by the first collision, and then again by the second impact.

"I felt the *twang* in my neck and knew I was in trouble," she recalls. "The headache came on fast and spread over the back and sides of my head."

Watson managed to drive her badly damaged car home. It was eventually written off by the insurance company.

"When I got home it really hit me," she says. "Every muscle in my body ached. The next day the headache was still there and I was very sore all over. I couldn't move very well. I went for a medical checkup and was given a neck brace and a prescription, Vicodin, a pain reliever. I really needed it There was no way I could get comfortable without some kind of medication easing the pain.

"On Christmas day, I met Dr. Jacob at a holiday gathering and he inquired about my situation. When I told him what had happened, he suggested I try MSM. I followed his suggestion. The day after Christmas I started taking MSM orally and had a friend apply the gel to my sore neck.

"I didn't like the bitter taste of the MSM, but I didn't want to be taking the drugs much longer. I have had a few surgeries in my life. I have used quite a few pain relievers and I know how easy it is to get used to them. After my whiplash injury, the pain relievers were really very helpful. But a few days later I wanted to move on and get started on something else.

"I am usually negligent about taking pills or vitamins, but I felt right away that the MSM was working for me. Within three to five days, I was getting significant relief. By the third day, the headache was a good 40 percent better. Within ten days I seemed to be my old self again. I was still a little sore and if I turned my head too fast, I would have a little pain. But otherwise the intense headache pain was virtually gone. And I have had no problem since. I have no doubt that the MSM got me through the whiplash fast. I really lucked out.

"My orthopedic doctor was very impressed with the recovery and just said to continue whatever I was doing as long as it is working."

Neck injury from a rear-end automobile collision often causes neck pain and whiplash headache that usually last weeks or months, according to experts. Headaches can sometimes last even longer before clearing up. Patients typically need painkillers, muscle relaxants, and physical therapy. Watson took a double hit and suffered a double whiplash, yet she says her headache started to diminish within hours after starting on MSM, and within two weeks it was gone.

Whiplash was first documented in the medical literature in

1886 and called "railway spine" in reference to train passengers facing away from the point of a railway collision. With the advent of the automobile, the incidence of rear-ending increased and by 1923 the consequences became known as "traffic light disease." Today, whiplash injuries are said to affect a million people each year in the U.S. alone and up to 40 percent of them develop chronic symptoms. High on the list of symptoms is headache.

Whiplash causes inflammation and muscles to spasm in the back of the neck, which in turn lead to headache in many cases. A physician can actually feel the tightness in the neck by palpating (pressing with fingers) over the affected area. After MSM is taken orally or applied topically as a gel or lotion, you can feel the muscles relax and the patient will say the tenderness has lessened.

If you are not taking MSM as a regular daily supplement, our recommendation is to start using it as soon as possible after a rear-end collision or any kind of injury from an accident. Our clinical experience indicates that you can reduce pain and lessen the severity of long-standing problems associated with the whiplash syndrome. Start with as high a dose of MSM as is comfortable. Apply an MSM gel or lotion topically. However, be sure to seek medical attention if you have sustained an injury.

Headaches from Chemical Sensitivities: Chris Dugan's Story

When Chris Dugan, 29, of Gardiner, New York, started a new job as manager of the supplement department in a health-food store she saw signs of trouble immediately. Dugan has suffered most of her life from chemical sensitivities. She is particularly bothered by chemical compounds in synthetic carpets and construction materials in new buildings. When she enters a new building her eyes start can start puffing up within minutes. She becomes dizzy and then headaches follow that may continue for a day or two or return intermittently for a month.

For two years, Dugan had been relatively headache free. Then she started her new job in a new store located in a newly constructed building.

"It didn't take long before I realized the new environment was going to adversely impact my life," she says. "The puffiness around the eyes started. I felt fatigue coming over me. I developed a headache. I know my body. I was reacting to the building. After a half-hour in the store I would be sick and just hold on for the rest of the day."

Around this time, Dugan started taking a gram of MSM three times a day, and then over time slowly increased her level to about ten grams.

"The first week I felt no difference," she says. "The second week I was feeling a little better. Less head pain and less fatigue. Then in the third week I realized at the end of my shift one day that the headache was gone and I actually felt quite good. I am now physically OK with the store and that's a surprise for me. I believe that if it hadn't been for the MSM I would probably have had to quit my job."

Chapter Nine

Fibromyalgia

"My gift from God":
Joyce Scott's Story

Joyce Scott, of Fountain Hills, Arizona, was as good as dead for five years.

"I used to be the most active person you could imagine," she says. "I had raised five children, did aerobics, and made and sold dolls out of my home. One morning after I returned from a doll show, I couldn't get out of bed. I was beyond exhaustion. I could hardly move. It came out of nowhere."

What came out of nowhere is what doctors diagnosed as chronic fatigue and later as fibromyalgia.

"I started to hurt around the clock and after a while the pain would wake me up at night," she says. "It would migrate all over my body and be worse at one time in my knee or in my shoulder or left hip or lower back. I had constant headaches. It was as if my whole skeleton hurt from head to toe. Even my fingers hurt, sometimes so bad that it took my breath away."

The 62-year-old Scott says that her condition also affected her clarity of mind. "I couldn't remember where the drinking glasses were in the house or how to drive to the bank and I have lived in the same place for more than twenty-five years. I stopped driving because of the mental confusion. If I had a good week friends would take me to play mahjong. Otherwise I was as good as dead for five years."

Scott took anti-depressants because she "didn't have a life anymore." But she says she couldn't take pain pills because they upset her stomach.

During her ordeal, friends were constantly recommending different supplements for her to take, including MSM.

"I am a very cautious person," she says. "I don't jump into everything. But I saw that a friend of mine with a candida problem had gotten relief taking MSM so I decided to try some myself. That was July of 1998. I didn't like the taste much, but things started to happen right away so I stuck with it."

Scott says she has had a rosacea condition and it started to clear up within days. Rosacea is a chronic red coloration affecting the skin of the nose, forehead, and cheeks.

"That was the first thing," she continues. "Then the energy started to kick in. During the second week I had one bad day but I felt I was getting better, and by the third week I had so much more energy.

"The pain started gradually going away, and after three weeks there was considerable relief. Now, a month and a half later, I am pain-free most of the time. That's why I call MSM my gift from God.

"I have a pool that is thirty steps down from my house. I have been in that pool more in the month and a half since I started taking MSM than during the previous five years. I can go up and down the steps with ease and go up the hill now to get my mail. I couldn't do that before. I'm driving again, and I'm living again. Now I feel good enough so that I am about to relaunch my doll business, which has been on hold for five years."

Scott says she started with a half teaspoon of MSM crystals with water in the morning and evening and then slowly built up to three teaspoons twice a day. As a result of feeling better she has started to reduce the amount of the supplement she takes.

About Fibromyalgia

Fibromyalgia is a relatively recent term for a common rheumatic disease that was previously called soft tissue rheumatism, fibrositis, or nonarticular rheumatism. According to the Arthritis Foundation, it is the second leading arthritis-related condition. The American College of Rheumatology believes 3 to 6 million Americans are affected. The Arthritis Society of Canada estimates the prevalence of fibromyalgia is between 2.1 and 5.7 percent of the population, with women affected four times more than men. The incidence increases with age and is said to be the most common in women 50 or older.

Common degenerative arthritis involves the joints of the body. Fibromyalgia attacks the soft tissue—the muscles, tendons, and ligaments. Symptoms include persistent burning, soreness, pain, and stiffness all over, a flulike feeling, headaches, irritable bowel, fatigue, insomnia, anxiety, and depression. The severity of symptoms fluctuates, but most patients experience discomfort on a daily basis and some pain is always present.

Fibromyalgia is hard to diagnose because many of the symptoms mimic those of other diseases. The American College of Rheumatology has developed certain diagnostic criteria. The main elements are widespread pain for a period of three months or longer, both above and below the waist, and on both sides of the body, as well as the presence of tenderness in at least eleven of eighteen specific, localized areas, particularly in the neck, spine, shoulders, and hips.

The cause of fibromyalgia is not known. Before symptoms develop some patients report having had a viral, bacterial, or parasitic infection, or a physical trauma such as an automobile accident, fall, or athletic injury. Among the possibilities are also poor diet, steroids, birth control pills, antibiotics, food allergies, nutritional deficiencies, and chemical sensitivities. Fibromyalgia may be associated with changes in muscle metabolism, such as decreased blood flow, which causes fatigue and decreased strength. Recent studies funded by the National Institute of Arthritis and Musculoskeletal and Skin Diseases also indicate an association with low levels of the anti-inflammatory hormone cortisol.

MSM cannot cure this major painful condition. But it is an excellent source of safe and substantial relief. Women diagnosed with fibromyalgia who have taken MSM say it has relieved their condition better than anything else they had previously tried.

This great benefit comes from MSM's pain reducing, anti-inflammatory, and increased blood-supply properties, but there may be other mechanisms at work that have yet to be determined.

Three More Cases of Relief

Case #1: Pain and Allergies . . . Both Gone

For Oregon businesswoman Gail Lind, allergy season is so traumatic that she moves to Hawaii for three months of the year to escape the pine and grass pollen.

"I don't just get the runny nose and eyes. I become extraordinarily nervous and fatigued," says Lind, 56, from Richland, Oregon. "The pollen literally puts me to sleep. It knocks me out."

Lind began taking MSM early in 1998 because she heard it helped allergies.

"It worked big time for me," she says. "This is the first time in twenty years I haven't had to remove myself from the pollen environment. I have had absolutely no symptoms. And this has been a very high pollen season."

Lind's story doesn't end there. Not only did she get total allergy relief, but the MSM erased the severe pain of fibromyalgia she had been battling for a year.

"The fibromyalgia was something new," she says. "It came on like a Mack truck in 1997 and just crushed me. I couldn't believe how severe it was. I am a pretty tough person but by three or four in the afternoon I was crying from the pain. It was wearing me out. It started in my neck, went down into my shoulders, and then within two months enveloped my elbows, wrists, hips, and my whole body. It was like something inside was twisting, pulling, squeezing, and crushing my body.

"The pain came and stayed and got worse with any movement. If I tried to lift my arms and rotate my shoulders it was as if thousands of little knives and pins were stabbing me. It was so bad I couldn't walk up the stairs. I had to think twice about driving anywhere because getting in and out of my car was excruciating. I am a very active busy person. I exercise a lot. This just completely put me out of commission. The pain took over all my thought processes. All I could try to do was work through the day."

Lind says she doesn't like to take medication, but out of desperation she got a prescription for Vicodin, a popular painkiller. It didn't help her. It was around this time that she started taking about five grams of MSM a day in an attempt to head off her annual allergy ordeal.

"I couldn't believe what happened," she recalls. "I wasn't expecting any pain relief, but overnight my pain was knocked down 50 percent. I literally jumped for joy because I could actually jump! As I continued to take the MSM, the pain became less and less. And now there is hardly any pain at all."

As her pain level decreased, Lind experimented with the level of MSM she required for complete relief. She found that thirty grams a day worked best for her.

Lind's experience is quite common. Lower levels of MSM frequently result in rapid improvement but to eliminate the most resistant pain you may have to raise the dosage appreciably. When you increase the dosage, always do so slowly. Mixing the crystals in water or other liquids is the most convenient way to take more of the supplement. Take it in divided doses during the day, preferably with meals. Always be comfortable with what you take. If you experience any gastrointestinal discomfort, reduce the dosage. See Chapter 3 for more details on how to take MSM.

"I need to keep my dosage at a high level, because if I don't I notice the difference," says Lind. "Some pain creeps back in. But I'm grateful because the MSM is really keeping the wolf from my door and giving me time to find the cause of the problem. I am out walking and jogging five miles a day now plus keeping up with a very busy business life. I am really amazed. I got a two-for-one-deal with the MSM. Both my pain and allergies . . . gone."

(Case #2:) "I'll see you next year."

Without assistance, Charlotte Callan, 72, of Burlington, Ontario, couldn't put on her own clothes, insert her arms into her coat, make the bed, or get in and out of the car or the bathtub. She couldn't put her hands over her head, and when she walked she was bent over. She had terrible pain and stiffness from fibromyalgia.

In 1988 her family doctor prescribed cortisone.

In 1996, a year after she started taking an MSM nutritional supplement, Charlotte was feeling so good she was able to stop the cortisone.

"I was glad about that because of the side effects from cortisone," she says. "The MSM worked well for me. I kept getting better and better. Now I can do everything. I have a little stiffness but at my age, you kind of expect that. If I sit for too long I can get a bit stiff. But nothing compared to what I had before. There is very little pain and a lot of energy. I don't even like to remember how bad it was. The MSM is pretty marvelous. I can do all the things now that I couldn't do before. It keeps my life worth living."

Callan takes about ten grams in her juice every morning.

"I go for my regular medical checkups and do the lab tests," she says. "They come out pretty normal. My tests for inflammation are normal. My rheumatologist looks at the tests, checks me over, and says, 'You have no swelling, no pain, no nothing. I'll see you in a year.' "

(Case #3:) "MSM reversed my direction."

"I basically was hurting all over all the time with throbbing pain," Barbara Redmond says, describing her ordeal with fibromyalgia.

Redmond, 40, of Lewisburg, Tennessee, was diagnosed with fibromyalgia in 1986. It came at a time in her life when she was raising two small children.

"My husband was taking care of a lot of things that I would normally do because it was so very difficult for me to function," she recalls. "If I did the dishes it would take two hours. I would have to go rest in the middle and then get up and finish them. I even had trouble combing my hair. I would get muscle spasms in my legs that were terrible. Walking was a problem, and sometimes I had to use a cane. I even had trouble speaking sometimes because the pain was so intense. It drained me. I just had to go to bed.

"It was so hard for my children to see me like that. My son, who was eight at the time, wanted to stay home and take care of me. The pain was so bad sometimes that I prayed for death to take me."

She took Elavil, an antidepressant, at night to fall asleep. She also used pain pills. Prior to her diagnosis of fibromyalgia, she had taken cortisone and gold for rheumatoid arthritis.

"I believe that all the medicines weakened me in some way and contributed to the fibromyalgia," Redmond says.

Redmond was luckier than most people who suffer for many years with fibromyalgia. Three months after her diagnosis she came to the Portland clinic and started a regimen of five grams of MSM daily.

"MSM reversed my direction," she says. "Within a matter of a week, I started to feel less pain and slowly regained my ability to function more normally again."

Along with the MSM she also did muscle therapy, slowly started to exercise, and watched her diet. She took pain pills if she needed them, which was mostly in the beginning. Sometimes if she had muscle spasms she would take muscle relaxants.

"But basically MSM has taken the pain down to a level where I can function again," she says. "It's down to about 10 percent of what it was before. I'm happy with that. I can take care of my family and do what I enjoy doing."

Today, Redmond works as an inventory specialist, a job that sometimes requires her to climb up and down ladders and audit inventory in large stores.

"I could never have done anything physical like that, but I can do it now as long as I keep taking the MSM," she says.

Chapter Ten

Muscle Pain and Athletic Injuries

"Bodies are just not made to put up with what we ask them to do."
—Dick Butkus, ex–Chicago Bears linebacker

About Muscle Soreness

Athletes and active people have countless ways in which to damage their bodies and cause pain.

There is, of course, the obvious risk of major injury to muscle, tendon, ligament, and bone associated with the very nature of sports and exercise—when you lift, push, pull, run, bike, jump, throw, hit, block, tackle, and kick hard enough.

Whatever the activity or sport, if it involves constant pounding and trauma, over time it has the potential to develop major injuries. The extreme effort and fatigue involved in endurance events, for instance, create a continual insult to tissue that may show up one day as painful leg or back problems. In addition, repeated micro-trauma to muscle tissue can accumulate and lead to strength-and-motion-limiting adhesions and scar tissue.

You may feel great after a major blasting of your musculature at the gym but the next day you may not be able to move a muscle without screaming pain. Those sore muscles are, in part, dead muscles. When you work a muscle too hard you damage and often outright destroy many of its fibers (cells).

Major muscles, receiving the brunt of stress, suffer the most damage. The punishment literally tears apart the fibers, releasing structural proteins and their amino acid components into the bloodstream where they become part of a circulating protein pool to be used for tissue repair and new muscle growth.

This painful consequence of all-out effort is known as delayed-onset muscle soreness (DOMS). Even weekend warriors experience it, as does the person who, after months or years of inactivity, jumps into an exercise program and overdoes it. Sure enough, the next day or two they are sore as hell. Deep down, the sudden or excess stress causes micro-trauma to the connective tissue—the cells and fibers that give support to muscles and organs. This damage releases a caustic enzyme that irritates local nerve endings and triggers pain. There is also localized rupture of tiny blood vessels and subsequent inflammation, adding to the discomfort.

MSM and Athletic Injuries

MSM is widely used by athletes, bodybuilders and fitness enthusiasts to reduce the pain, soreness, and inflammation associated with injuries, strained, or cramped muscles, and over-extended joints.

We have treated many athletes over the years who have often mentioned the problem of muscle soreness after workouts. MSM has helped many of them.

At the International Preventive Medicine Clinic in São Paulo, Brazil, Efrain Olszewer, M.D., and his staff treat many sports-related sprains and tendinitis.

"Usually we have treated these injuries with DMSO, which has always worked very well, but we find we get just as good results with MSM, which works without the DMSO odor," says Olszewer.

The Brazilian physician often gives his patients an MSM ointment that a pharmacist prepares specially for him. He directs patients to use the ointment twice daily on the affected area of the body.

"Sprained ankles, elbows, shoulders, tendon injuries, and muscle soreness all respond excellently," says Olszewer. "The normal pain, inflammation, and reduced function of the area of the body all appear to be reduced significantly."

Most of these injuries he treats involves fitness enthusiasts, weight lifters, and martial artists, says the Brazilian physician. Some older people who have over-extended themselves benefit similarly from the MSM.

Four Cases of Relief

Case #1: Quarterback Aches

June Jones, the former Atlanta Falcons quarterback and presently head coach of the San Diego Chargers, has used MSM and says it helps reduce the aches and pains from old football injuries.

"All the aches and pains in my fingers, hands, elbow, and shoulders subside," he says. "I just put the crystals in juice and it makes me feel like a well-oiled machine."

Case #2: Sore Feet

Business lawyer Joe Durkee, 29, runs two or three long-distance competitions a month for the "Red Lizards," a Portland athletic club. Marathons and triathlons are his specialty—long, grueling, punishing events.

Durkee has been at it for years and routinely trains hard, including a minimum of eight miles a day running in a hilly urban park. The constant pounding has created a chronic soreness in his feet, particularly on the heels and balls. Runners commonly get this condition—called plantar fasciitis.

"Originally, I used to ice my feet but the effect would not last long. The pain would come on again soon," he says.

Then Durkee discovered MSM. Three times a week he soaks his feet in a foot bath of warm water with about sixty grams of dissolved MSM for fifteen to twenty minutes. "It eliminates the pain quite effectively and gives a lasting effect," he says.

Durkee also takes about eight grams of MSM orally.

"I'm a real MSM junkie," he says. "I keep it in the shower and gargle with it if I ever feel a sore throat coming on, which occurs from time to time after hard training or competitions. If I actually develop a sore throat, I will gargle several times a day. And it just gets rid of it. I am amazed. If I am congested I swab my nasal passages. It eliminates any congestion. It works great."

Durkee's experience with sore throats is not unusual for many athletes or exercise enthusiasts who put extra high demands on their bodies. Exercise done at a nonexhausting level enhances the immune system. But too much is depleting. A drug works the same way. A little bit may be beneficial. Too much can make you sick or even kill.

Some years ago researchers conducted an experiment with laboratory animals. In the study, one group of rodents were run to exhaustion and a second group was given a less demanding challenge. Afterward, all animals were exposed to a virus. The results: Rampant infections among the first group and an increased resistance among the second.

MSM can be helpful not only to stave off the muscle soreness and pain that often results from overtraining, but also to fortify the body against colds and flu that are known to plague the finely tuned bodies of high performers.

Although we don't know the precise mechanisms involved, MSM appears to exert a positive, normalizing effect on the immune system, including some protection against the garden variety of colds and flu. Many patients have told us that after starting to take MSM they aren't as cold-prone as they used to be.

(**Case #3:**) Knee Pain

Physical therapist Frank J. Smith, 46, was having difficulty walking up the one flight of stairs to his office, the Canwood Family Physical Therapy and Sports Medicine Center in Agoura, California. His knee was often in pain, a result, he thinks, of years of pounding long-distance running when he was younger.

Anti-inflammatories had helped, but he was wary of them because of the side effects he had heard about.

The pain in his knee would intensify whenever he overdid the exercise demonstrations he gave throughout the day for his patients.

Smith had tried a variety of supplements over the years but with little effect. One day a patient told him about MSM, and although he was skeptical, he started taking it.

"Around my house I'm a Mr. Do-It-All," says Smith. "On the weekends I enjoy painting, gardening, and plumbing and keeping the house in shape. Increasingly I was noticing that on Mondays I would be sore all over, tired, and almost in a flu-like state.

"Immediately after starting the MSM this feeling disappeared. No soreness. No fatigue. I would take it Sunday night and wake up on Monday feeling great.

"As I continued taking the MSM I noticed that the pain in my knee was decreasing. I was no longer limping into my office just from walking from the parking lot, up a slight incline to the building, and then up the one flight of stairs. Moreover, I was now able to do much more exercise in the clinic with patients without fear of the knee hurting me.

"Another bonus is that the fatigue I usually felt at the end of my working day wouldn't develop if I took MSM in the afternoon. I found I could stay up later at night and get up earlier feeling very refreshed."

Smith says the MSM has rehabilitated his knee to the point where he now gets out with his teenage sons, shoot hoops, and fools around with the football, without any pain.

"Before, I couldn't do that, or if I did, I had to be very respectful to my knee and not overdo it," he says. "Now I can really challenge the boys."

(Case #4:) Shin Splints

Maggie Fredericks, 19, is a heptathlete at Ball State University in Indiana. Heptathletes are all-around athletes who compete in the high jump, long jump, shot put, javelin, 800- and 200-meter runs, and the 100-meter hurdles. Jackie Joyner-Kersee, the great American Olympian, is a heptathlete. The combined events put great stress on the body.

In Frederick's case, her intense workouts caused painful shin splints to both legs. Shin splints are inflammations of the muscles on the shins. The standard prescription is ice, massage, pain relievers, and rest, ideally sitting out days at a time to allow your legs to heal. But even after the rest the pain often comes back, particularly if you train at a level of high intensity.

"I got shin splints so bad in high school that I had to sit out most of my entire last year of track competition," says Fredericks. "In college, the problem has continued, and being involved in multiple events makes it very difficult to miss practice. I have just had to tough it out and bear the throbbing pain in my legs, which was pretty constant after workouts."

That was before MSM.

"It has made a huge difference," she says. "Once you have shin splints you always have them. But I started feeling relief within two weeks, and after one month I was almost pain-free despite quite hard workouts. It also relieves many of the minor muscular aches and pains. A friend of mine on the track team also started using MSM, and it helped her muscle soreness as well as a problem with cold sores."

Fredericks takes one gram of MSM a day. She says that she ran out of MSM at one point, and her shin splints started gradually returning. After resuming the supplement, the symptoms of pain vanished again.

Recommendations

As a general rule, follow the suggested range of dosage (see Chapter 3). If that relieves your muscle soreness there is probably no need to take more. Many athletes and bodybuilders involved in intense training are taking relatively high amounts of MSM before and after workouts and report that it greatly diminishes or eliminates the usual soreness. If you still experience soreness following workouts or events, you may want to slowly increase the dosage before or after to see if the extra MSM provides additional relief. If you have any doubts about how much to take, always start with a small dose and increase slowly. Taking too much MSM at one time may cause minor stomach upset or headaches.

MSM and Weight Training

The following report is based on the experience of one well-conditioned athlete who follows a high-intensity training program. The level of MSM he uses may or may not be appropriate for you.

Scott Magers, 34, of Irvine, California, is a personal trainer and former high school and collegiate baseball coach who lectures widely on nutrition to bodybuilders and athletes. He has been using MSM for nearly a year.

"I have trained with weights since 1979 at a very intense level and there has never been a time after doing heavy leg work that there isn't some stiffness and soreness the next day . . . until MSM came along," he says. "After only a day or two, I experienced a significant decrease in muscle soreness. This great benefit has continued and at this point I regard MSM as the most effective supplement I have ever taken—and I have taken a lot of supplements.

"As a result of not having the soreness, I have been able to increase the intensity of my training even more, including my cardiovascular training. I run every other day and the stiffness and lactic acid buildup from my weight lifting is just not there anymore.

"The MSM has reduced the usual after-effects so significantly that sometimes I feel I haven't even worked out. I squat three hundred and ninety-five pounds, do lunges and dead lifts. I am training at a very intense level so for me to notice as significant a change as this—that is, no soreness—has been the biggest breakthrough in all my years of weight training.

"Usually when you do your rep sets, you have a burning feeling as you get to the fourth, fifth, or sixth rep, but even that has diminished significantly. The burn is from the buildup of lactic acid. As a result of not having that burn, you can do an extra rep or two.

"I have recommended MSM to many athletes, and the feedback has been consistent. Aches and pains in the knees, shoulders, or other joints are greatly diminished. Delayed-onset muscle soreness is greatly reduced. Any effect of the lactic acid cycle is lessened and you are free to workout the next day."

Down in your "engine room"—the billions of muscle cells throughout your body that contract to create motion—an exquisite ritual of biochemistry takes place.

Adenosine triphosphate (ATP), an organic compound that is the body's main source of energy, is used up quickly when you start exercising, necessitating muscle cells to create more ATP from glycogen (stored sugar). When this occurs, lactic acid is produced. As it accumulates, it retards the contraction process. At this point, oxygen enters the picture to rescue the wilting muscle cell. Oxygen combines with lactic acid to produce glycogen, which is then converted to ATP. This biochemical sequence permits indefinite contraction provided that sufficient oxygen is available.

In sustained intense activity, however, the circulatory system cannot supply enough oxygen. The lactic acid builds up to cause fatigue, muscle pain, contraction shut down, respiratory distress, and a reluctance to continue.

Magers recommends MSM for both elite athletes who are pushing themselves as well as for weekend recreational types who "won't have to face the usual day-after soreness, or at least have much less of it."

Magers says that some of the athletes who have started on high amounts of MSM develop a slight headache after two or three days but then "they feel great."

He reports that some athletes who previously were taking steroids or other drugs have become sick for a day or two after starting a high dosage of MSM.

"There may be some detoxification process going on," he suggests.

Magers, at 5-foot-10, 195 pounds, and 6 percent body fat, says one other thing about MSM has impressed him: "My skin. It's become smooth, clear, and almost baby soft."

Magers says his normal dosage of MSM is 3 to 5 grams (3,000 to 5,000 milligrams) of MSM just before and after a workout. He increases the level on days of particularly heavy lifting.

"This is what works very well for my body but may not be appropriate for the next person," he points out. Many athletes and bodybuilders are taking higher than usual levels of MSM, he adds.

"With most supplements I've taken over the years I could never tell the difference," says Magers. "With this one, I can tell a difference."

"MSM Soaking" for Athletes

In the chapter on osteoarthritis, we mentioned a promising use for MSM as a hot-tub soak to relieve pain. Dick Brown, Ph.D., of Coburg, Oregon, one of the premier track and field coaches in the United States, has been exploring the soak concept for athletes as well. He feels it offers "tremendous potential" for speeding muscle recovery from hard training and as a preventive and therapeutic aid against injury.

"It appears that MSM is able to soak into the skin after a period of time, saturate the tissues, and reduce the inflammatory process," he says.

Brown has experimented with the idea by setting up an inexpensive model of a hot tub an a health spa, filling it with 140 gallons of water maintained at 94 degrees, and then adding 315 pounds of MSM crystals.

He then selected ten individuals—half of them track athletes and the others fitness enthusiasts—to soak in the tub for up to one hour five days a week for six to eight weeks. The participants had a variety of common training-related complaints, such as plantar fasciitis (foot injury) and knee injuries.

"My observation is that this method is effective," says Brown. "Pain and inflammation are reduced. It appears that if there is a specific injury, the soak will shorten the recovery time and lessen to some degree the severity of the injury. Obviously, some injuries are severe enough to require surgery. But if you strain a muscle or develop a tendinitis, the difference between soaking and not soaking may be substantial."

Brown also feels that the MSM can make a significant contribution to an athlete's recovery time from hard training.

"When people are working out hard, they often do not understand that they have to balance the challenge of their physical exertion with the body's recovery process," he explains. "Recovery involves a lot of things. When are you really improving? You are improving or adapting only when you are in the recovery mode. Challenge simply tells the body it needs to improve. Anything you can do to enhance recovery, such as eating properly, obtaining enough rest, and probably soaking in that tub will enable you to recover from the challenge of workout much faster, and your potential for injury will be decreased. If you are hurt, getting in the tub will hasten the recovery from the injury."

Brown feels that professional sports teams should investigate the potential of soaks for their high-priced and often-hurting athletes.

"After a workout, an athlete sits in the tub for fifteen or twenty minutes or even ten minutes," he says. "There is a temporary relief of pain for some hours after the soak. But I believe that when the soak is repeated over days and weeks, the MSM will build up and stay in the system, continually modifying the injury. Such tubs would be like bringing healing sulfur springs right to the training facility."

What's the difference between the MSM soak and a regular hot tub? A hot tub can only be used after the acute phase of an injury has passed. But an injured athlete can use an MSM soak immediately after an injury since the water is below body temperature.

Moreover, a hot tub "wilts you" while an MSM soak, he believes, has a relaxing, stress-reducing, and restorative effect. He has observed that soaking in MSM, no matter what time of the day it was done, enhanced relaxation and sleep. The participants in his experiment also commented that their skin had become smoother.

Brown also sees a potential use for MSM soaks in hospitals and rehabilitation clinics for enhancing healing from injury in general.

Brown admits that his experience is limited: "I haven't done controlled scientific studies, looking at specific injuries and how MSM benefits them compared to people with similar injuries who don't use the soak. But what I've seen so far is impressive and leads me to believe that studies should be funded and carried out."

Chapter Eleven

Tendinitis

MSM is a valuable natural remedy against most inflammatory musculoskeletal conditions involving the tendons and ligaments. Many of these problems are caused by repetitive and stressful motions related to work or sports. According to the National Center for Health Statistics, about four million workers suffer from tendinitis.

Forceful, repetitive motions can create damage and inflammation of the tendons connecting muscle to bone or the ligaments connecting bones and cartilage. Injury to these tough cords of fibrous tissue may result in severe pain, chronic soreness, scar tissue and stiffening, and loss of movement.

MSM provides effective relief for such problems as the following:

- Tennis elbow (also known as pitcher's elbow or bowler's elbow)
- Golfer's elbow
- Tendinitis of the shoulders, arms, legs, and feet
- Achilles tendon contraction
- Bursitis

We have found that in general 6 to 8 grams a day of MSM orally helps reduce the pain and swelling. Some people find that less is also effective. Others need more. For additional benefit, rub a 15 percent MSM gel or cream over the affected area several times a day. Healing time is faster if you use MSM both orally and topically.

Back to Pain-Free Massages: Pekka Mero's Story

Pekka Mero is a 6-foot-2, 195-pound massage therapist who specializes in that most physical of massage techniques, deep-tissue massage. It's hard work, like kneading wads of clay. You manipulate layers of muscle to get to the deeper layers of soft tissue beneath in order to relieve soreness, tension, and fatigue. You use a lot of pressure but at the same time you use special strokes so that you don't cause bruising.

Mero lifts weights and stays strong to meet the challenge. He has been doing it for nearly twenty years but can't put in more than twenty hours a week without his hands, wrists, and forearms becoming sore.

Recently, the soreness at the end of a long day had turned into pain that sometimes kept him awake at night. Mero, 42, from Calabasas, near Los Angeles, was forced to modify some of his techniques because of the tendinitis he had developed in his forearms.

"I was just not able to do all my usual strokes without causing more pain," he says.

Mero tried anti-inflammatory medication, which dulled the pain but didn't take it away. So he stopped the medication. Then a friend told him about MSM. He took a teaspoon of crystals twice a day in warm water. Two days later more than half of the pain was gone.

"After a particularly hard day with five massages there was

only twenty-five percent of the pain that had been there only a few days before," he says.

Over the next few days, the remaining pain continued to disappear. His ability to rotate his wrists was easier. He could put his usual pressure back into his strokes.

After ten days, the pain had become "almost nonexistent," he says. "The stuff really works."

Back to Pain-Free Shoveling: Ken Miners' Story

Ken Miners, 53, of Burlington, Ontario, developed a persistent tendinitis in his elbows after hours of shoveling gravel to make a driveway for his cottage getaway. He had had brief episodes of muscle soreness from physical exertion in the past but this time the pain was severe and continued for months.

"This time both elbows became stiff and painful and remained so for months," he says. "Bending them caused more pain. The bony part on the outside of the elbows became inflamed and if I bumped my elbows going through a doorway, for instance, it was quite excruciating. The pain was sometimes bad enough to keep me awake."

Miners, a water researcher, learned about MSM from his wife who was taking the supplement for relief of her back pain. Within a few days of starting the supplement, he noticed a reduction in the pain.

"Within three weeks the pain was completely gone, and my normal mobility was restored," he says. "Now, some soreness may develop with prolonged heavy shoveling or exertion, but it is relatively minor compared to before and it always subsides within a day or so." Miners takes a teaspoon or two of MSM crystals on a regular basis.

Back to Pain-Free Running:
Dan Drown's Story

In the summer of 1997, Dan Drown decided to challenge his body on a twenty-five-mile circuit of a steep Yosemite mountain trail. The 56-year-old California lawyer, a former U.S. Olympic water polo star, keeps himself in top shape with a regular running routine and didn't expect any problems.

On the descent, however, his legs gave way.

"I didn't realize how exhausted my legs were from the steep climb up and the pounding going down," he says. "I had to use two walking sticks and frequently sit and rest."

At one point when Drown rose to his feet after resting he toppled over and realized he had hardly any muscle strength left in his legs. Afterward he rested standing up and gritted out the remainder of the trail to the bottom.

"I thought I was in good shape but hadn't realized that a steep climb such as this was extremely punishing to the legs compared to flat running," Drown says.

Except for two days of soreness, he experienced no other ill effects and felt comfortable about doing another vigorous, though shorter, hike two weeks later. Apparently the original trauma had not healed and the physical stress of the second hike caused substantial aggravation and inflammation in the tendons, tendon sheaths, and ligaments of both knees.

"The pain came on strong this time and went on for four months," says Drown. "I couldn't walk or run for any distance at all and even had extreme difficulty standing up in the morning. I started to live on aspirins in order to be able to function. I took two in the morning and two more in the evening. If I didn't take them, I couldn't walk. I went from someone running thirty miles a week to someone who couldn't walk to the mailbox."

When Drown made an appointment to see one of us (Lawrence) he was recommended to try MSM.

"I followed the advice," says Drown, "and the next day later I felt a substantial difference. After two weeks all the pain was gone and I was able to start running again. I took two heaping tea-spoons three times a day in the beginning. And then I cut back to one level teaspoon twice a day."

Drown says he stopped the MSM for a short time and noticed the pain returning.

"Now I find that I am OK if I take it every day I run, and I usually run about four miles five days a week," he says. "If I am not running I take it three or four days a week. My knees are not like they used to be, but I can still run. There is no pain anymore but when I run I do feel a little stiffness. But I am grateful for the relief."

Ronald Lawrence, M.D., Comments:

One recent case involved a 16-year-old boy who injured the ten-dons behind the knee while playing soccer. Usually, an injury like that for someone his age would take ten days to two weeks to heal, using a combined approach including ice and/or moist heat and magnetic therapy. With the addition of MSM, the youngster was fully recovered in a week and back on the playing field.

He took three teaspoons of MSM daily.

I have found that about 60 to 70 percent of my patients with simple bursitis or tendinitis respond very well to MSM.

Stanley Jacob, M.D., Comments:

Epicondylitis is an inflammation of the lower end of the arm and the tendon near the elbow, usually a repetitive strain type of injury, and can be extremely painful. I have treated the most seri-ous epicondylitis patients and there is rarely a quick fix for these very severe types of inflammation, which can sometimes take a year or more to heal. You may start to see some symptomatic relief with MSM topically and orally within a few weeks but don't expect to eliminate this severe problem overnight. Any signs of early relief are likely associated with the involved tendon. Soft tissue responds faster than the hard tissue of the bone. True epicondylitis may involve inflammation of the lower humerus, the bone above the elbow, and it is in this area where pain can persist. You have to give it time. Physical therapy, cortisone, and acupuncture are often used, but no matter how you treat the problem, it takes time.

Chapter Twelve

Carpal Tunnel Syndrome

About Carpal Tunnel Syndrome

Carpal tunnel syndrome is the most widely reported repetitive strain injury (RSI) that occurs in the workplace. RSIs affect the hands, arms, shoulders, necks, and backs of workers who do the same repetitive motions for many months or years. Such motions include gripping, twisting, bending, lifting, reaching, cutting, and keying.

The National Institute of Occupational Safety and Health (NIOSH) says RSIs have increased in recent years because of automation and job specialization where a given job may involve only a few manipulations performed thousands of times per workday.

Carpal tunnel syndrome is named for the eight bones in the wrist—the carpals. They form a tunnel-like passage filled with tendons that control finger movement and the median nerve that carries nerve impulses to and from the hand. Repetitive flexing and extension of the wrist may cause an inflammation of the protective sheaths surrounding the nerve, which produces symptoms.

Generally, the problem first appears as painful tingling in one or both hands during the night. Most commonly, the thumb, index, and ring fingers are affected. Later, tingling can develop during the day, along with a decrease in dexterity and grip power.

Women, according to Bureau of Labor statistics, account for nearly two-thirds of all work-related carpal tunnel conditions and repetitive strain injuries even though they comprise only 45 percent of total employees.

Deborah Quilter, author of two books on the subject, including *The Repetitive Strain Injury Recovery Book* (Walker & Co.), says the reasons for greater female susceptibility are these: a narrower carpal tunnel, smaller and weaker muscles than men, as well as hormonal changes from pregnancy, menopause, and gynecological surgery that can contribute to swelling.

"The higher proportion can also be attributed to the large number of women in jobs that require repetitive movements of the hands and arms, such as data entry operators, telephone operators, and cashiers," she says.

Prevention and symptom-reduction strategies include redesigning tools and tool handles to enable a workers' wrist to maintain a more natural position, modified layouts of work stations, and special exercises that include simple flexing and extending of the wrists, turning the head from side to side, and yoga postures.

At the first sign of symptoms, "see a competent physician immediately," says Quilter.

It is interesting to note that over the years medical researchers have found that many carpal tunnel sufferers have a variety of concurrent medical conditions. Diabetes, thyroid disease, wrist osteoarthritis, and any form of inflammation affecting the wrist joints or tendon sheaths have been frequently associated with carpal tunnel. Some researchers suggest that health factors, and not just occupational activity, may promote or aggravate symptoms. In a 1998 study in the *Archives of Internal Medicine* a group of researchers found that 40 percent of 213 patients with carpal tunnel had a metabolic, inflammatory, or degenerative condition "that might have caused the symptoms." Nevertheless, they noted, a direct cause-and-effect relationship to carpal tunnel has not been proven.

Conventional treatments for carpal tunnel involve wrist braces, anti-inflammatory medications to reduce swelling, and steroid injections. If these fail, several different surgical procedures are available to relieve pressure on the median nerve. Such treatments, however, "have met with mixed results, especially when an affected person must return to the same working conditions," according to NIOSH.

MSM and Carpal Tunnel Syndrome and Related Problems

We see many patients with severe carpal tunnel. Often they have already been operated on before, sometimes even twice, and still have the same discomfort, pain, and disability. Frequently the problem is worse afterward. We have not been impressed with the surgical approach to this condition.

We believe that oral and topical MSM can be as good as any conservative approach. Approximately 70 percent or more of the individuals who take MSM regularly report significant reduction of pain.

Improvement may come quickly or may not become significantly noticeable for a couple of months, depending on the severity of the condition and whether the person is continuing to aggravate the wrist.

One woman who started taking MSM for muscular aches and pains reported that her carpal tunnel–related pain started to diminish within a few weeks and then "disappeared." We can't say the MSM will cause carpal tunnel to disappear, but it should help in many cases to ease the level of pain.

MSM can be beneficial in a number of ways. The two key points are these:

- MSM reduces inflammation. This property is important because any inflamed tissue in the wrist may impact the median nerve running through the carpal tunnel. Such inflammation may be caused from occupational tasks performed repeatedly, or, as suggested earlier, created by an underlying inflammatory condition.

- MSM reduces pain.

In addition to these effects, MSM may also help by increasing the blood supply to the area and softening scar tissue surrounding and compressing the median nerve.

Pain Gone . . . Energy Restored: Sue Ellen Andrus' Story

Despite her small stature, Sue Ellen Andrus, a businesswoman in Montrose, California, has always been proud of "keeping up with the guys," as she puts it.

"I've always been competitive, an outdoors and physical type with lots of energy," she says. "Over the years I have enjoyed using my hands swinging a sledgehammer, bailing hay, driving tractors, chopping brush, or just helping friends with remodeling work."

Several years ago, Andrus' strong hands began to rebel.

"They first started to become numb, and later they began to hurt," she says. "The pain would bother me the most at night, and sometimes the pain would wake me up. I also developed an achiness in my forearms."

Andrus had also lost her normal energy and become chronically fatigue.

"I would wake up tired, have energy for an hour or so, and then feel wasted. I needed to nap two or three hours and would still feel wasted. My mind had become foggy. Mentally and physically, I was out of it and really worried," says Andrus.

In early 1997, an acquaintance told Andrus about MSM.

"I started taking a half a teaspoon of the powder twice a day in orange juice, and I was pretty amazed because the next day I had more energy and could breathe better," she says. "I was excited but cautious because other health products had given me an energy boost in the beginning too and then sort of faded out. Much to my amazement the energy never left. Over the next few weeks my fatigue was improving and I no longer had to take long afternoon naps. And above all my mental clarity has returned."

It was sometime around two months after she started taking MSM that Andrus noticed one day that her wrists and hands were not bothering her.

"There was no more pain and no more numbness," she says.

Andrus has continued taking MSM and one-and-a-half years later says her energy level has remained high and she has had no more pain in her hands.

"I have my hands and my energy back again," she says.

Amazing Relief of "Trigger Thumb": Alondra Oubre's Story

Alondra Oubre, Ph.D., is a medical researcher in the San Diego area who had developed a painful, debilitating tendinitis of her hands. Her thumbs were particularly affected. She was diagnosed with "trigger thumb," also known as DeQuervain's tenosynovitis, a type of tendon injury. The problem had intensified over more than two years to the point where it seriously affected her ability to use the computer keyboard in her work.

"Sometimes in the morning the thumbs would be locked straight or bent so rigidly that I would have to put my hands in hot water to release them," she says.

Oubre had undergone surgery on one hand, received steroid injections a number of times, but still had recurrent pain and disability. She wanted to avoid nonsteroidal anti-inflammatory drugs because of their notorious side effects. She had taken an array of supplements, homeopathics, and topical analgesics. She felt she was getting reasonable relief, particularly from the homeopathics and topicals, that allowed her to slightly push her time on the computer.

"I was still limited," she says. "If I overdid it, I would pay for it with pain."

An acquaintance told Oubre about how MSM had helped his shoulder tendinitis.

"I began taking 750 milligrams of MSM twice a day," she says. "After three or four days, I noticed improvement. After a week, the relief was significant. After two weeks, it was amazing. I had had some relief before with all the other remedies I used, but the MSM took the relief up to a new level. I now have whole days without any pain at all. The relief is such that I don't think I will require any more injections. That's what I am hoping for. Now I am able to use the keyboard with at most minimum pain. I just take a break whenever the pain comes and it goes right away."

Chapter Thirteen

Temporomandibular
Joint Syndrome (TMJ)

About TMJ

Press a fingertip into the flesh just in front of the middle of your ear and open and shut your mouth a few times. Feel the joint moving? That's the temporomandibular joint (TMJ), the hinge that allows you to open your mouth, bite, chew, talk, and shout. Your finger is on one of the most strategic joints in the body, a major nerve junction to and from the brain, and also a major trouble spot for nearly 30 percent of the population, according to the American Dental Association.

TMJ Dysfunction or TMJ Syndrome, as it is known, involves a wide array of potentially debilitating symptoms that are produced when the jaw joints do not work together in synchronized harmony. Symptoms can range from a dull ache in front of the ears to devastating pain and dysfunction throughout the body, says the Jaw Joints & Allied Musculo-Skeletal Disorders Foundation of Boston, a nonprofit educational organization. The foundation says that TMJ is "one of the most pervasive, least understood and controversial health disorders in existence today."

Clicking and grating the joints, inability to open or close the mouth freely, and difficulty in chewing and swallowing are often evident.

There is little consensus at the present time about treatments, symptoms, and causes, the organization points out, yet millions of Americans complain of dysfunction or pain in the head, face, jaw, neck, and shoulders that are indicative of TMJ. In addition, seemingly unrelated problems such as back pain, leg cramps, and nausea can be attributable to TMJ.

Pain and dysfunction may be "temporary, chronic (continuing for longer than six months) or intractable (never ending)," says the foundation.

Most frequently, TMJ dysfunction is said to be caused by malocclusion (improper fitting together of the teeth and jaw joints), arthritic changes, trauma such as whiplash or a blow to the head, poor dental work, and stressful grinding of the teeth or clenching of the jaws. In the case of Linda Dickter, it was probably bruxism, a lifelong involuntarily grinding of her teeth at night.

Singing the High Notes Again:
Linda Dickter's Story

In 1994, when she was 56, the pain started on the left side of her face. It got to the point over the next year and a half where she had to limit her diet to baby food, well-soaked cereal, or very well-cooked vegetables because chewing anything harder would cause excruciating pain.

"If I ate a salad or even chicken I would pay for it," she says.

Specialists said her problem was synovial chondromatosis with calcified floating bodies, one of the most severe of TMJ disorders. In layman's terms, it means that the years of hard grinding pressure on her teeth had deteriorated the cushioning material in the jaw joint and, in addition, small chunks of hard calcium had formed. Visually, there was a protrusion the size of half a Ping-Pong ball in front of her left ear.

"I was in agony any time I opened my mouth and even when my mouth was closed I had pain. There was no time of the day that I wasn't in pain. I was often awakened in the middle of the night by terrible pain," says Dickter, who teaches English as a Second Language to adults in Brookline, Massachusetts.

Dickter made the rounds of doctors, looking for relief and answers. Specialists couldn't help much except to prescribe anti-inflammatories, which didn't help and made her sick. Pain relievers, along with acupuncture four times a week, helped to make the pain partially bearable.

TMJ problems often respond to chiropractic, but a chiropractic physician examined her and said her situation was too severe for his method. A dental surgeon suggested removing the soft tissue in the joint and then creating a hinge from muscle tissue taken from elsewhere on her face. Dickter checked out the surgical track record for her condition and found that most of the operations done were to repair previous surgeries.

"It was not a statistical revelation that inspired confidence," she says. "I passed."

At her night school classes, Dickter's ability to teach suffered drastically. She had to explain to her students why she often had difficulty opening her mouth to speak with enough energy so they could hear her.

"I did my best," she remembers. "My pain would increase over the two hours of teaching. I would suffer through the pain and then go home, apply an ice pack, and often take medication as well."

Her singing also suffered. Dickter is a first soprano in a Brookline choral group that performs at a semi-professional level at local venues. First soprano means singing the highest notes. As she tells it, when you hit a high note you have to open your mouth wide for maximum effect. But she could barely open her mouth without incurring excruciating pain.

"I thought I might have to drop out of the group," she says. "I certainly couldn't open my mouth properly to sing. I continued to do the best I could. My conductor and fellow singers were very understanding. I had to try to move my mouth in a way that didn't kill me. As hard as I tried, it was still agonizing and I would sometimes have to leave for the restroom to douse my jaw with cold water."

A tip from her acupuncturist prompted Dickter to look into MSM. She found out that one of us (Jacob) was speaking in Pennsylvania and traveled there, accompanied by her daughter, to learn more about MSM. As a result of that meeting she was encouraged to start a program of oral and topical MSM.

Slowly she began to feel improvement. "It was no magic wand," she says. "It took time. The pain slowly started to diminish."

After a few months, Dickter was talking and eating more comfortably. Within a half year she believes the pain level was down to about a quarter of what it had been before. The swelling was mostly gone in almost a year.

"In just over a year I was able to eat like a normal person again," she says. "Today, in 1998, I am for the most part pain-free and have no significant discomfort as long as I take the MSM. If I forget to take it for even a day or two, I begin to feel discomfort returning. The physical condition is still there. But the pain is largely gone and I have my life back."

Recovery extended to her singing life. As her condition improved, she could once again move her mouth properly to handle the most demanding high notes. She recalled one transcendent moment during a performance of the Bach Cantata No. 191 in D major: "I can't forget it. At the second I hit the high note I felt the music as an electric charge that enveloped me from head to toe. As that note vibrated within me, I realized there was no pain. I could sing with no pain."

MSM can work well for TMJ problems. Use it orally as a daily supplement and apply the gel or lotion to the affected joint. It acts as an anti-inflammatory and analgesic, softens scar tissue, increases blood supply, and reduces muscle spasm. If it can help Linda Dickter's problem, which is as bad as it gets, it can be of help to other sufferers of TMJ.

Relief for Dickter means taking a high level of MSM—about forty grams a day. Most patients are not as severely affected and do well with much smaller doses.

Chapter Fourteen

Dental Pain

If you have dental pain, see a dentist. MSM probably isn't going to eliminate your problem, but it may help the healing process and provide some relief of pain and inflammation.

We believe that MSM offers an additional weapon in the fight against gum disease, a problem that affects 75 percent of Americans over thirty-five years of age.

Gingivitis is an inflammatory condition of the gums that can be aided by MSM. If neglected, gingivitis turns to periodontitis, which means progressive infection, more inflammation, loss of the tiny ligaments that bind the gums to the teeth, bone recession, and loose teeth. Whatever you are doing for this condition, add MSM.

MSM crystals or capsules can be used "straight," just as you would take any nutritional supplement by mouth. Follow the general recommendation of two to eight grams daily.

To benefit oral health directly and help lessen the inflammation caused by plaque activity, you can also use MSM as a mouthwash. See Chapter 3 for directions on how to mix MSM crystals and water. Swish the mixture in your mouth two or three times daily.

MSM may also provide benefits when applied directly to the gums. Many patients have told us they have helped lessen the inflammation of gingivitis by repeatedly rubbing MSM crystals onto affected gum tissue.

We would like to recommend that dentists look into the value of MSM as an oral and topical addition to their regular treatment.

MSM and Tooth Sensitivity

MSM can help dental patients with tooth sensitivity, according to Craig Zunka, D.D.S., a holistic dentist in Front Royal, Virginia.

"After you have worked on somebody's teeth, such as fillings or crowns, the teeth are sometimes sore and the nerves are hypersensitive. MSM reduces this soreness and calms the sensitivity," says Zunka.

"Apply the MSM directly to the gums. Open a capsule, pour the contents onto a small plate, and add a bit of water to make a paste. Rub the paste on your gums over the root of the sore tooth. Some of the MSM appears to be absorbed right into the tissue. The rest dissolves in the mouth."

Zunka says that more than fifty of his patients have used this simple method and reported less discomfort. He suggests applying the paste in this manner twice a day for a day or two after treatment.

In Spartanburg, South Carolina, John L. Tate, D.D.S., recommends 3 grams of MSM daily to his patients to help with inflammation, recovery of teeth following dental work and reduction of tooth sensitivity.

"I find it very beneficial for patients who have had a lot of dental work and who in general have more tooth sensitivity," says Tate. "The MSM brings the inflammation rate under control in the dental pulp (nerve), which reduces pain and sensitivity. This also reduces the risk of future root canals, in my opinion."

More on the MSM—Tooth Sensitivity Connection

● Teeth with gold inlays can sometimes be a source of pain and sensitivity to heat or cold for a long period of time after the dental work has been performed. A dentist can reduce the risk by simply applying a small amount of a 15 percent MSM solution onto the tooth surface prior to inserting the inlay.

● Similarly, a 15 percent solution or some MSM crystals can be applied to the gum socket immediately following a tooth extraction. This will help prevent "dry socket" sensitivity in the area. The patient can also apply topical MSM to the external surface or the cheek or lower jaw adjacent to the site of an extraction. This will help lessen inflammation and reduce pain.

Healing on Two Fronts

We recently spoke to Margaret Itow, an eighty-year-old Los Angeles grandmother, who patiently used MSM to heal a stubborn and painful infection involving three of her teeth.

Here's her story: "Three upper teeth had become infected and very painful. They were teeth on which I had had root canal work done about twenty-five years ago. The teeth throbbed and kept me awake at night. My dentist gave me an antibiotic to relieve the infection and recommended I see a specialist, an endodontist. But I was reluctant to have surgery. The antibiotic worked as long as I took it, but the pain returned after the medication wore off. The same thing happened two more times, and then I developed thrush.

"Around this time I happened to notice that my mechanic, who has arthritis and is unable to walk comfortably, was dashing around without any apparent pain. I asked him what had happened. He told me he was taking MSM. I had never heard of MSM but because I had a painful, arthritic finger, I asked him if he had any information. He gave me an article as well as a generous amount of his own MSM crystals for me to try. In the article I read a story about a woman who healed pyorrhea with MSM. I decided to try to heal my infection with MSM as well. I took three tea-spoons of the crystals daily, and in addition I applied the crystals night and day to my gums."

We spoke to Itow six months after she started using MSM regularly in this fashion.

"Each day there was less pain and inflammation. Within two weeks I was able to sleep much better," she said. "The infection kept getting progressively better. Now there is no pain. It healed!"

What really surprised Itow was what happened the second day after she started using the supplement. She woke up to find that the pain in her finger was gone. Three years before she had devel-oped arthritis in the first joint of her right index finger. The finger had become severely painful and bent at a thirty-five degree angle.

"It was giving me pain every day," she said. "I used to ice it and then soak it in hot water but it didn't help much for the pain. But then two days after I began taking MSM the finger was straight and no longer painful. It was unbelievable."

MSM and Tooth Whiteness

As we age, so do our teeth. In the process, they tend to become darker. Several patients have mentioned that brushing with MSM made their teeth whiter. Our curiosity was aroused and so we asked some patients to try it. The feedback has been positive.

Give yourself about two weeks to start seeing whiter teeth. First do your regular daily brushing. Rinse off the toothbrush. Then put some MSM crystals on the wet brush, enough to cover the top of the bristles. Before brushing, allow the crystals to soften further and dissolve on the brush inside your mouth. Then brush as normal. Do this once or twice a day.

MSM has started to appear as an ingredient in toothpaste.

MSM and Lichan Planus

This condition involves a hardening of the mucous membrane tissue of the oral cavity. Again, create a mouthwash with the MSM crystals and swish it in your mouth two or three times a day. You should see improvement within several months.

Chapter Fifteen

Heartburn and Hyperacidity

About Heartburn

You chew and swallow, and if all is well the mush balls of food drop straight down the esophagus and into your stomach for digestive processing. If all is well . . .

Heartburn is that burning sensation felt in the upper chest or lower neck area that is sometimes misinterpreted as a heart attack. Often it is a sign of gastro-esophageal reflux disease (GERD), a chronic condition that allows acid from the stomach to rise upward into the esophagus and sometimes as far up as your mouth. The incidence of GERD, and the heartburn it produces, is often underestimated, according to experts, who say that as many as a half of patients with unexplained chest pain, chronic hoarseness, or asthma may be suffering instead from this condition.

GERD may occur as a result of weakness in the valve at the bottom of the esophagus that is designed to prevent just that from happening. The feeling of heartburn can be associated with inflammation and bleeding in the esophagus.

Symptoms usually start within an hour of eating.

Esophageal reflux may also be related to a hiatal hernia, a

bulge of the stomach through a hole in the muscular diaphragm separating the abdomen from the chest.

Many of us have occasional heartburn, but frequent heartburn may be a sign of GERD and should be brought to the attention of a physician. Approximately 10 percent of Americans experience heartburn on a daily basis, and many of them turn to over-the-counter preparations such as Pepcid, Tagamet, and Zantac.

About Hyperacidity

When food enters the stomach, it gets a dousing of hydrochloric acid (HCL) and pepsin, a digestive enzyme. This chemical activity breaks down protein and prepares the food for the next stage in its digestive processing in the small intestine.

If you overeat, consume too much fried and fatty foods, overdo it with coffee, and you smoke, you run the risk of producing too much acid in the stomach. Over time, constant hyperacidity, in combination with a specific bacterium called helicobacter pylori, can cause the development of stomach or upper intestinal ulcers. The regular use of nonsteroidal anti-inflammatory drugs, often prescribed for arthritic conditions, is another major cause of ulcers. The common symptoms of ulcers are heartburn, burning or pain over the area of the stomach, and pain while lying down or during the middle of the night.

Standard medical treatment for ulcers includes antacids, bland diets, antibiotics, and anti-ulcer drugs. Although some of these measures can be effective on a short-term basis, relapses frequently occur.

Stanley Jacob, M.D., Comments:

In 1982, after using MSM in my clinic for a few years, I made the following brief comment in a report for the Annals of the New York Academy of Sciences: "Subjects seen to be chronic users of various antacids and histamine H2 receptor antagonists prefer

MSM by reason of relief obtained coupled with freedom from serious, untoward effects." (H2 antagonists are acid suppressant agents).

In the ensuing years, patients have continued to tell me that they find MSM gives them relief from heartburn comparable to such medications as Tagamet or Pepcid. These are individuals who have been taking antacids and anti-ulcer preparations.

Based on clinical observation, the use of MSM frequently permits a patient to lower the dosage of stronger prescriptive medication. It helps to relieve pain and discomfort in many cases.

MSM may offer anti-ulcer potential and be a useful adjunct in the treatment of gastric acidity disorders. The precise mechanism for its effects in this area are unknown at this time. We need studies to determine these important details.

My son Stephen developed GERD and used MSM to wean himself off Prilosec, a powerful gastric antisecretory agent. He was diagnosed in 1997 after complaining of stomach pain and severe heartburn that would frequently wake him in the middle of the night. Any food he ate could cause the problem, but it was more likely to happen if he ate too much, too late, and finished off his meal with ice cream.

Prilosec worked well for him. He didn't want to take it continually so he took MSM one day and the medication the following day. The combination was effective. After a short period of time, he was able to stop Prilosec totally and remain symptom-free by taking MSM every other day while eating an earlier and lighter dinner. Now he can even eat ice cream without a problem.

Ronald Lawrence, M.D., Comments:

Constant suppression of acid in the stomach with drugs is not desirable. I speak from personal experience. I have a congenital hiatal hernia with accompanying GERD. I have had to take Zantac on and off over the years, and on occasion, have taken Prilosec, the much stronger antacid.

Much to my satisfaction, I found that taking MSM has greatly relieved the pain and heartburn I have frequently experienced. Because of my personal interest in this problem I have mentioned MSM to patients of mine who have complained of frequent heartburn. A number of them who started taking MSM have told me they are able to reduce the use of acid-suppressing agents.

But MSM by itself is not a solution. Nor is Zantac. Nor is Prilosec. You must do other things. You need to look carefully at your diet and at what and when you are eating. For my own health situation, I eat a modified diet with six small servings a day. Eating small amounts of food at a single sitting makes a big difference. I also avoid tomatoes, tomato sauce, and citrus—all acidic foods.

Part (**THREE**)

How **MSM**

Helps Relieve

Your Allergies

Chapter Sixteen

Pollen Allergies

An Olympic Performance:
Jeff Roake's Story

Remember the 1996 Olympic Games in Atlanta? The weather was oppressive—blistering heat, smothering humidity, and plenty of pollen in the air to make life miserable for allergy sufferers like Jeff Roake, the official announcer for the cycling events. Roake, 47, is the "voice of North American cycling" and works the major racing events. He has had allergies since childhood.

"Athletes and Olympic staffers alike were wilting," he recalls. "But I had my secret cocktail to keep the allergies at bay, my energy high, and my voice strong."

Roake's secret is MSM. For particularly demanding events, he prepares an MSM "cocktail" beforehand. He dissolves MSM crystals in a thermos of hot water and adds freshly squeezed lemon juice. He gargles with the mixture several times a day and then downs the liquid.

"Some days, I had to announce for three or four hours in the morning and then come back for another three or four hours later in the day. I was fine, despite the elements."

Roake says he couldn't have done it without MSM.

"I'm allergic in a major way to so many things," he says. "You name it. I'm allergic to it. Acute sensitivity to dog and cat hair, to house dust, to wool. Seasonal pollen allergies. All of it.

"At the age of twelve I went to see a specialist, and he informed me that I had a big allergy problem. I didn't need him to tell me that. I would often wake up with a scratchy throat and clogged sinuses. Or I might have a full-on attack where my nose would leak nonstop like a faucet. I would be in total misery for hours. Pollen season would make my usual discomfort even worse.

"The doctor prescribed the usual medications and I took them all. The antihistamines would make my nose and throat irritatingly dry, and sometimes I would feel even worse. If I took any medication in the evening I would feel knocked out the next day. After a while I just limped through life with allergy problems and tried to avoid taking medication unless I absolutely needed it.

"In 1981, my mother told me about MSM. She worked for Dr. Jacob. I started taking the crystals off and on that year but not regularly. I took about a gram a day when I remembered. After several months, though, I noticed that my condition had improved to the point that it became clear the MSM was helping. I wasn't doing anything else different. So I just made a point to be regular."

For the most part, Roake has taken his MSM regularly ever since.

"There were some times over the years I ran out of MSM. If I didn't get a new supply of it quick enough, within four or five days I would start to feel my sinuses becoming uncomfortable and my eyes would start to run," he says. "I would just try to make sure I had a supply on hand so I didn't have to go through the torture again. And now, with Buddy, Fifi, and Blake sharing my household, I can't take any chances."

Buddy is a short-haired cat. Fifi is a very long-haired cat. Blake is the family dog.

"Fifi is all over me sometimes," says Roake. "Before MSM I wouldn't have been able to be in a room frequented by a cat, even if the cat wasn't there at the same time I was."

Roake credits MSM for keeping him strong and fully voiced each year when he worked the "Tour duPont," a major fourteen-day cycling event on the East Coast with leading European racers that was held between 1989 and 1996.

"This was a major challenge not just for the cyclists in the race but for the public-address announcer as well," says Roake. "It was seventeen days of all-out, high-volume, constant talking. In marathon events like this, the quality of your voice naturally drops over time, and you become quite fatigued. Once, one of the Italian team doctors asked me how I kept my voice strong. I told him about MSM. He was surprised and mentioned to me that one of the leading European cycling announcers protected his voice by taking steroids. I had heard before about rock singers taking steroids to keep their voices strong."

On demanding days, or when ever he feels the slightest "allergic twinges" in his nose or sinuses, Roake doubles his dose to about two grams. Otherwise, he keeps his allergies under control with one MSM cocktail every morning.

"I don't think the MSM has cured anything, but it's hard to imagine my life without it," says Roake. "I have to keep taking it to realize the benefits. I don't even like to think about having to get up every day and not having it."

About Allergies

You are considered allergic if you have an adverse reaction to a substance that is normally harmless to most people.

Such reactions can take all kinds of forms and are generated by all kinds of substances, including food, chemicals, and elements in the environment.

Symptoms include:

- Headaches
- Fatigue
- Sneezing
- Watery eyes

- Stuffy sinuses
- Mood and behavior changes.
- Diarrhea
- Coughing
- Skin rashes
- Muscular aches and pains

According to the National Institute of Allergy and Infectious Diseases, allergies are among the major causes of illness and disability in the U.S. As many as 40 to 50 million Americans are believed to be affected by allergies. Nearly 35 million people alone suffer from upper-respiratory symptoms that are allergic reactions to airborne pollen. Pollen allergy, commonly called hay fever, results in 8 million doctor visits a year.

Many physicians, such as Doris Rapp, M.D., author of *Is This Your Child's World?* (Bantam), specialize in environmentally induced illnesses and believe that allergies or sensitivities can strike anywhere on, or in, the body. They don't think that allergies are just limited to hives, hayfever, and asthma.

Sensitive individuals can develop an endless combination of mild to severe behavioral, emotional, and physical problems because of exposure to chemicals, pollen, dust, mold, food, and other environmental elements, claims Rapp.

"Anything is possible," she says. "When the nervous system and brain are affected, people experience a wide variety of psychological and behavioral problems. They may become violent, depressed, suicidal, exhausted, or unable to learn, talk, or write coherently. They may also experience headaches, muscle aches, menstrual problems, and urinary problems.

Such sensitivities are not generally accepted as allergies by traditional allergists. As a result, many patients fall through the cracks. Many are referred to psychologists or psychiatrists. "Unfortunately, these problems are often misdiagnosed and treated incorrectly," says Rapp.

Why does one person develop sensitivities and not the next? Much has to do with your genetic make-up. That may be the biggest factor. But it's not the whole answer.

The "barrel concept" helps to explain our individual vulnerability to allergies. Imagine your body as a barrel that can hold a specific amount of stress and pollution. Each person's barrel has a different capacity, depending on our genetic inheritance, so to speak.

If you are exposed to a small amount of dust and mold, your barrel has the capacity to hold it. But if on another occasion you are exposed to too much of any one or more pollutants, your barrel may overflow. When that happens, you develop symptoms.

Rapp and other environmental-medicine physicians believe that stressful lives, nutritionally poor diets, and the proliferation of chemicals make people more vulnerable. In other words, these factors shrink the barrel. It takes less stress and fewer contaminants to set the stage for reactions, which then occur earlier in life.

"We live in a time when our bodies have been exposed to an unprecedented onslaught of chemicals that are weakening our immune systems," says Rapp. "If this had happened over hundreds of years, perhaps humans could have adapted. Unless our nutrition is good we can't hope to detoxify these things. But our nutrition has deteriorated over the last half century and we are no longer the robust, hardy people we used to be. We never had as much cancer as we do now. We never had Alzheimer's. We didn't see babies you couldn't breast feed. Teachers will tell you they never had the behavioral problems years ago they are now having. The food we eat is processed, pesticided, and poor in nutrients. What we drink is full of chemicals. The result is that our bodies have become toxic dump sites and we are reacting quicker and more intensely to all the poisons and allergens."

Emotional stress can negatively affect your immune status and also shrink the capacity of your barrel. We know that many people with heightened allergic responses often have emotional problems. A constant barrage of anxiety and stress depletes the body's resources and resiliency and increases susceptibility to fatigue, allergies, and illness. Studies show that emotionally "stable" people seem to have a more robust constitution and better resistance to allergies. Emotional stress thus has the potential to undermine the body as would any devastating toxin or allergen from the environment.

When the body senses an allergenic substance, it goes into a protective and defensive mode. An enemy has been sighted, so to speak, and so the body summons its defenders. Among its reactions is the production of antibodies to combat the detected offenders. Certain cells throughout the body called *mast cells* release histamine, a secretion that triggers an inflammatory tide. Small blood vessels are dilated to make them more permeable to white blood cells, frontline "soldiers" of the immune system, which then can rush about engaging and neutralizing particles of allergenic material that have entered the body.

This scenario is part of the body's wondrous immune response. But there's a downside. For many people the release of histamine sets off precisely the symptoms associated with allergies. The small blood vessels leak and ooze fluid, causing a swelling of tissue around them.

The nasal obstruction in hayfever, for instance, comes from leaky vessels and swelling in the nose. Leakage and swelling in the brain can lead to malfunction among nerve cells and possible changes in mood.

Standard treatment for allergy involves antihistamines to neutralize the body's response. Such medicines can cause side effects, including the production of more histamine by the body.

Antibiotics, often prescribed to suppress symptoms, may unleash a whole array of new problems and even additional allergic reactions.

MSM and Allergies

When MSM was first being used for patients, primarily for musculoskeletal and other pain problems, a Portland area equine veterinarian named John Metcalf, D.V.M., became interested in the supplement. He was familiar with DMSO and had used it extensively in his practice. He now wanted to determine if MSM had any possible effects for unhealthy and chronically sore horses. But first he decided to evaluate the effect of MSM on his own allergy problem. He described his experience in a 1983 issue of "Equine Veterinary Data," a newsletter distributed to horse doctors.

"Much to my surprise," Metcalf wrote, "I found that my allergy problem was helped and that I had freer breathing. I had been through allergy testing some months before and was found to have a severe allergic reaction to just about everything having to do with the horse, including the horse itself. Since my practice is limited to horses, this allergy was a significant problem. After starting to add MSM to my diet, I felt better than I had in years.

"Not convinced that my improvement was attributable to MSM, I withdrew the MSM and returned to the earlier antihistamine therapy. My condition deteriorated. I again began to add two grams of MSM to my daily diet as a split dose and rapidly improved."

Feedback of a similar nature from patients soon made it clear that MSM was extremely beneficial for allergies. Patients would repeatedly say that their chronic allergies had greatly improved. These were frequently people with a lifelong problem and for whom medication had provided only limited relief.

The comment of one female patient years ago became something of an "allergy theme song" at the DMSO clinic. "I started taking MSM for my arthritis," she said, "and before I knew it my sneezing and coughing and allergic symptoms cleared up. You can't believe what a wonderful surprise this has been for me. This is the first time I can really say that my allergy is under good control. I wanted to share the good news with you."

For allergy sufferers, MSM is *very* good news. After many years of treating pain patients with MSM, it has become clear that perhaps the single most powerful benefit it offers is quick relief of the symptoms of common allergies. In hundreds of cases, this nutritional supplement has proved highly effective.

Severe pollen allergies can be incapacitating. You sneeze nonstop. Your eyes burn from morning until night. Antihistamine medications may or may not help. The impact of MSM on pollen allergies is so superb in so many cases that it just might be the best remedy since the advent of antihistamines a half-century ago.

People frequently say they have better results with MSM than with antihistamines. It works for people of all ages, from small children to centenarians.

In a great many cases, significant improvement comes rapidly, usually within a day or two, even for people suffering from allergies for years. Even before you find your most effective individual dosage, you are most likely already experiencing some relief. Not only do the characteristic congestion, sneezing, tearing eyes, coughing, and sinus symptoms improve, but other seemingly unrelated problems caused by allergies may also benefit.

MSM often enables people to reduce their allergy medication significantly and in many cases discontinue it. However, if you are on medication and under a doctor's supervision, do not change your medication unless consulting first with your physician.

In allergies, symptoms are related to inflammation and immune weakness. MSM is beneficial for both of these areas. MSM's action is not as an antihistamine substance that inhibits histamine production. Rather, we attribute its effectiveness to blocking the receptivity of histamine in sensitive tissues, such as the mucous membranes of the nasal passages. This action is something like shutting the cell door and preventing entry to histamine. This blockadelike action prevents histamine from creating inflammation, swelling, and fluid build-up. We don't know the precise mechanism involved. We do know that the observations and reports of relief are real.

MSM may also have a role by providing needed sulfur for the production of antibodies that the body uses to combat germs and allergens and the production of enzymes that counteract inflammation and promote the repair of damaged cells.

Stanley Jacob, M.D., Comments:

I have seen hundreds of allergy cases clear up with MSM, including my own. Years ago, I experienced the typical miseries of a seasonal grass-pollen allergy. From mid-April to mid-July, I required the usual antihistamine relief. In those days, the antihistamine medications often created a side effect of drowsiness. Today, they are less likely to do that. But way back then, it was a price you paid for relief.

If I didn't take medication, my eyes burned, my nose ran, and I developed nasal congestion, making it difficult to breath through my nose. Often the symptoms would persist throughout the day.

I started taking MSM more than twenty years ago, and it relieved my problem entirely. No eye irritation. No runny nose. No congestion. No problem at all through allergy season. I have continued to take MSM for all these years and have not had to resort to an antihistamine even once.

In the beginning I used MSM in the capsule form, taking two or three 750-milligram capsules in the morning and the same dose in the evening. Later, I took the same amount of MSM but found it easier and more effective if I mixed the crystals in a small amount of water. The dosage I need now to control my pollen allergy is one gram morning and evening.

My son Stephen, who is now 46, developed severe pollen allergies about ten years ago at just about the same age that I did. His hayfever came on so strong that he had to take time off from work. Stephen had constant sneezing. His eyes reacted terribly. When this happened, I recommended he start taking MSM.

Stephen says the following about his experience with MSM: "I took about a gram. Within a few days there was a marked decrease in severity, and my condition continued to get better, although I was never completely free of symptoms. After that I started taking MSM every year from the middle of May through July. I could basically control the symptoms although sometimes the pollen was so bad that I had severe attacks and couldn't work.

"In time I learned that if I started taking the supplement well before the start of allergy season and also doubled the dosage I could get even better control. I now have about 65 percent relief, I would say. Even this past season, which was extremely dry in Portland, I did quite well. I haven't had to take any time off from work for about four years thanks to MSM. I know I would do even better if I increased the dosage but when I do I get some intestinal reaction. My father and a lot of other people I know can take much more than I can. That's just my particular comfort zone."

For some individuals, 1 or 2 grams twice daily may be enough to bring pollen allergy symptoms under control. Others may require 3 or 4 grams twice daily. In general, relief is usually obtained within a range of 2 to 8 grams a day. Always start with a lower amount of MSM, and increase your dosage slowly to avoid the possibility of gastrointestinal discomfort. Should you develop any discomfort, such as increased or loose stools, just reduce the dosage.

For the common pollen variety of allergy you may not need a very high dosage. In some resistant cases, you may have to double the dose, and even double it again. Do this slowly. When you reach the effective level, you will notice rapid relief of allergic symptoms.

I have often been asked the question, "What if I keep increasing the dosage, and the allergic symptoms don't go away?" My answer is always the same: "Nobody bats a thousand." It just doesn't work for every person. But it works for many. In pollen allergies it works for most.

For best results, take the MSM in divided doses during the day. My recommendation is to take your doses in the morning and early evening. The evening dose is important because pollen tends to accumulate in the nasal passages at night and thus upon awakening you experience sneezing, coughing, and burning eyes. MSM taken in the evening will often prevent this from happening. But don't take it too late. It may give you energy and keep you awake.

Chapter Seventeen

Asthma

A Bad Day Turned Very Good:
Katherine Dubik's Story

On May 2, 1998, Katherine Dubik was having a bad day and not looking forward to the days that would follow. The weather was unseasonably hot. Allergy season was beginning, and her asthma was starting to make life miserable for her as it did every year at this time.

The 38-year-old Wilkes-Barre homemaker has suffered with asthma since the age of 5. She would routinely take three puffs from her home inhaler four times a day and carry a "rescue" inhaler with her wherever she went in case of breathing difficulty. She frequently had to use the emergency inhaler.

"Allergic reactions make my asthma worse, and I am allergic to grass, pollen, and tons of things," she says. "Late fall and winter, when it gets cold, I am better, but otherwise there is something out there that bothers me every season. Spring and summer are particularly bad."

On May 2, Dubik was feeling the itchiness around her eyes and was already wheezing more than usual. As she walked up the steps to her front door after returning from church, she was disgusted and discouraged: "Here we go again, I was thinking. More wheezing, congestion, itchy eyes, sinusitis. Another great allergy season in the making."

Dubik lay down on the couch, breathing with difficulty.

"I'll just try those dumb pills," she said to herself. She opened the bag she had carried into the house with her, pulled out the plastic bottle, opened it, and took two capsules. The bottle contained MSM. A friend had just given it to her and said it might help her.

"I had gotten to the point where I would try anything," she says.

Dubik speaks in tones of amazement when she recalls what happened next: "I remember looking over to my husband, and asking him how long I had been lying there.

" 'Twenty minutes,' he said.

" 'Guess what,' I said to him. 'I can breathe again. My lungs feel so clear. This is impossible.' I had never felt so much air. And in such a short time I was breathing comfortably and no longer wheezing. It can't happen that fast and from some nutritional supplement. But it did happen. And I have continued to experience relief as long as I keep taking the MSM."

After three weeks Dubik saw her doctor for a checkup, and he couldn't hear a wheeze inside of me.

"He couldn't believe it either," she says. "Several months before I had been to see him with acute sinusitis and asthma. With this turn of events, he now thought I could stop the regular inhaler, but he advised me to still carry the 'rescue' inhaler just in case."

When we talked to Dubik, four months after she started MSM, she hadn't had to use her inhaler a single time.

"My breathing is good and I sleep like a baby," she says. "Previously, I would frequently wake up wheezing in the middle of the night."

Once she ran out of MSM. It was sold out in all the stores she visited. It took three days before she found a source, and in that time she started to struggle again with her breath. After resuming the MSM, she once again experienced ease of breathing within twenty minutes.

Dubik started on 4 grams a day for 2 weeks. Then she took 6 grams for another week, and then increased her dosage to her present level of 10 grams.

"Not only am I breathing and moving around so well, but I just went through a very bad pollen season with no problem at all," she says. "Many people I know were complaining about their allergies. For a change I wasn't complaining. I am amazed. MSM is the only thing I am doing that is different."

About Asthma

For most of us, breathing in and breathing out is an automatic, background activity in life. But for asthmatics, breathing in, and particularly breathing out, is no mindless matter. Asthma is an inflammatory condition of the bronchial tubes, the passages that carry oxygen into the lungs and gaseous waste products out. The airways become inflamed and spasm, excessive amounts of clogging mucous develop, and muscles surrounding the airways become constricted. In acute asthmatic episodes, breathing becomes so labored and difficult that the condition becomes as life-threatening as any killer disease.

Asthma afflicts so many people that medical authorities describe it as an epidemic. About 15 million Americans suffer with the condition and 5,000 die each year, double the rate of twenty years ago. The American Lung Association estimates that there are 3.7 million youngsters with asthma, an increase of 200 percent over the past twenty years.

Asthma is the most common chronic illness of childhood, affecting about 10 percent of youngsters. It is widely thought of as a condition you outgrow. While symptoms often diminish after childhood, the problem can recur when people reach their mid-twenties. Today, in fact, asthmatics over the age of fifty are at the highest risk.

Airborne allergies to pollen, mold, animal dander, and dust

mites are often involved in asthma and can exacerbate the condition. Food allergies and chemical sensitivities may also be contributing factors.

The standard medical treatment for asthma has for many years focused on symptom-suppressing drugs known to cause side effects. Bronchodilaters (inhalers) are used to expand the airways. Anti-inflammatory drugs (oral pills and inhalers) target the buildup of mucous. The effectiveness and safety of these drugs have been widely questioned. One 1992 study declared that regular use of bronchodilators may actually increase the risk of dying from asthma! Other studies indicate that children on asthma drugs have a slower rate of growth.

In 1997, the *New England Journal of Medicine* published a study indicating that asthmatic children using the steroid inhaler experienced a slightly reduced rate of growth. The youngsters were following the recommendations and rinsing their mouths, gargling, and spitting after the inhalation of the dry-powder medication. Yet enough medication appeared to be absorbed that affected their growth. More recently, a new generation of drugs have appeared that block the action of leukotrienes, biochemical agents involved in the inflammatory process of asthma.

Stanley Jacob, M.D., Comments:

Severe asthma can be an incapacitating illness for many people. We have seen at least a dozen children with severe enough conditions that they had to be hospitalized for a good part of a year. They couldn't go to school. They were being maintained on huge doses of cortisone. While these drugs are important agents for many illnesses they have severe downside potential.

One such child was a five-year-old girl with visible signs of cortisone toxicity. She had a moon face and was developing a hunchlike condition of her back as a result of the changes to her bone metabolism. Her growth pattern was also disturbed. Because of extreme difficulty breathing she had been hospitalized for two-thirds of the previous year.

The girl was started on MSM and over a one-month period was slowly brought up to eight to ten grams per day, given in divided doses. Her mother mixed the MSM crystals in water, juice, or any beverage that the girl enjoyed drinking. For the following two months the level of cortisone was gradually reduced, and then the drug finally stopped. The girl's asthma was not cured with MSM, but her symptoms were largely relieved. She attended school the next year without missing a single day. She has now been maintained solely on MSM for five years and plays and interacts with other children in a normal fashion. She has had no side effects from the MSM.

Physicians don't particularly like to give children cortisone. Once the MSM begins to take effect it may be possible to start lowering the cortisone. This should be done only under the guidance of a doctor. Whenever cortisone is taken orally or intranasally, your adrenal glands stop producing the natural cortisone hormone, cortisol, which is essential for life. By gradually reducing the intake of cortisone you give your body a chance to gear up and start producing its own cortisol. You do not want to stop cortisone suddenly. There are tests that your doctor can do to determine if your body is producing cortisol.

We find that we can wean children off cortisone and sustain them with MSM alone. This is not possible with an antihistaminic agent. Asthmatic children usually do not need more than eight grams a day, although some resistant cases have required higher doses. Start with about two grams daily, in divided doses, and increase if needed.

We have treated several dozen asthmatic adults with good results. Most of these are individuals under fairly good control with cortisone medication. With the addition of MSM we can reduce the requirement for cortisone to the extent that the patient no longer experiences any of the adverse side effects from the drug. Adults usually require more MSM than do children for control. Also start at two grams and increase slowly as necessary.

After Ten Years—Time for a Refill:
Joyce Jensen's Story

Joyce Jensen, 57, manager of a research facility storeroom in Portland, hoped that she would be just as lucky with MSM in 1998 as when she first took it more than ten years before. In the late 1980s, she developed allergies, asthma, bronchitis, and a continual low-grade fever.

"Nothing would help me," she recalls. "Any medication I took just bounced me off the wall or made me drowsy."

Jensen heard about MSM while working at Oregon Health Sciences University. She obtained a supply of crystals and to her surprise, "it worked like a miracle."

Within a few days, Jensen says, her health started to improve and her symptoms eventually cleared up. For a couple of years she took a quarter teaspoon of crystals (about one gram) each morning in orange juice. Then she stopped.

For years, she had no problem. Then in 1998, she transferred to a new work location, and the symptoms returned. She thinks it had to do with working in a dust-filled environment.

"I started having allergic symptoms again and difficulty breathing," she says. "I was very sick three times this past year and once I was out of work for a week and needed to use inhalers. Basically I was feeling icky most of the time."

Then Jensen remembered MSM. Could the magic work the second time around? One week after she started back on a quarter teaspoon she reported major improvement.

"It was pretty amazing," she says. "It did the job again. The sneezing and runny nose are gone. I still have a little cough and a little drainage, but I feel so much better. Plus I have a lot more energy. I feel like a new person."

Jensen says this time she isn't going to stop the MSM.

Her case is interesting in that she experienced relief from symptoms for years even after she stopped taking MSM. Many people find that when they stop the supplement their symptoms return. The MSM may have produced a substantial long-term healing effect in her body that was finally overwhelmed when her new job environment exposed her to more dust than she could handle.

No More Asthma Attacks:
Lauro Scozzaro's Story

Laura Scozzaro is a licensed practical nurse working at the Center for Nutrition and Digestive Disorders in Hanover, Pennsylvania. In 1997, she moved from Florida to Pennsylvania. That's when she started having asthma attacks.

"I had gone from the city into a country setting and into a brand-new house," she says. "Whenever I would dust in the house, the asthma would suddenly flare up. I would have real difficulty breathing. I always thought that dust was dust. There is plenty of dust in Florida and I never had a problem.

"But the attack could come any time. Perhaps from the pollen in the air, cat dander, or something else in the new environment. It was terrible. Whenever it happened, my chest would start tightening up. I would gasp for air. It was scary."

Scozzaro started using Primatene Mist, an over-the-counter inhalant that gave her relief. The spray would open up the airways.

"There were days when I was using it four or five times and I began carrying it with me all over because I was afraid of having an attack at any moment or any place," she says.

When Scozzaro started taking MSM, the asthmatic symptoms vanished.

"One time I ran out of MSM and I didn't get a new supply," she says. "I thought I would see if it was all in my head. It wasn't. I started having problems again. I also noticed a muscle achiness in the morning that wasn't there when I took the MSM. If ever I miss a day or two taking the MSM, I start having allergic symptoms such as post-nasal drip and nasal congestion. When I resume the MSM, everything is fine again, and overall I just feel better."

Scozzaro says she takes a teaspoon of MSM once a day in the morning with juice.

Ronald Lawrence, M.D., Comments:

Primatene Mist or other sprays are useful for symptomatic relief, but many asthma specialists say that if you need to use them more than once a day you should probably be on a prescription medication. The problem with all these preparations, whether over-the-counter or prescription, is that they tend to drive blood pressure up to some degree and may cause nervousness. Every asthmatic I have spoken to tells me that they feel some edginess or irascibility after taking medication.

From personal and clinical experience, I regard MSM as an exciting new option against asthma. As a youngster, I had a minor asthma problem related to sinus and post-nasal drip conditions. For many, many years I had no significant symptoms, even after I started running marathons at the age of 41.

In 1991, at the age of 65, I was flying to Boston to participate in the Boston Marathon when I suddenly experienced an acute asthmatic attack—the first really serious episode in my life. It could have had something to do with dehydration in the interior of the plane or the quality of the recirculating air.

At any rate, the incident kicked off the problem and I have been fighting it ever since with every medication and supplement available. At times it was so bad that I had to use inhaled steroids two or three times a day.

Once I was hospitalized for three days, not because of the asthma per se but because of my reaction to medication. I had gone to the emergency room of a nearby hospital after my breathing had become particularly difficult. The attending physician, a young doctor, said he was going to give me an injection of Benadryl, an antihistamine. I questioned him about the rationale, but he insisted it would help. It helped me right into the hospital with an acute asthmatic episode.

Following this incident, I did some research and found out

that antihistamines, for the most part, are counter-indicated for asthmatics. These types of medication dry mucous membranes, thus interfering with the normal lubrication of the airways and the ability to clear out congestion.

Antihistamines are indicated for allergic conditions. Asthma is now recognized as primarily an inflammatory process. It often has allergic elements to it, but antihistamines can frequently make the asthma worse and should be used with great caution.

This is where MSM is so good because MSM helps both the asthma and allergies. I started using MSM about two years ago. After two weeks I found that I was breathing much easier. In a short period of time I found that my forced expiration volume (FEV) had improved about 70 percent. FEV is a measurement obtained from a peak flow meter, a handheld device used by many asthmatics. It measures your bronchial output—that is, your ability to breathe out, which is the primary problem with asthmatics. I am amazed at how my FEV readings have maintained this substantial level of improvement since I started taking MSM. Normally, as you age, you lose lung capacity, even if you don't have asthma or any respiratory problem.

I still enjoy running several miles a day and take one quick whiff of the inhaler as a precautionary measure. I believe this is advisable for any asthmatic running long distances or exercising intensely. But the MSM on its own has made a big difference in my breathing comfort zone when I am out running and with the normal muscle soreness that develops afterward.

In my neurology practice, I have a number of patients who also have asthma. I have told them about MSM and their feedback has been very positive. One of them is a woman in her mid-forties whom I have known since she was nine years old. When I first saw her, she was taking steroids for her asthma. I started treating her then with acupuncture, which worked very well, and she was able to stop the medication. Many cases of childhood asthma can be helped with acupuncture, along with drinking plenty of fluids, keeping the air filtered at home, and trying to avoid allergens. In her case, she had been doing well and I would see her maybe once a year for a recurrence related to a flu or cold. She, like all asthmatics, has a diminished FEV. After starting to take MSM she also experienced a 50 percent increase.

There are a number of basic things that asthmatics should do to help reduce their symptoms.

Asthmatics frequently have minor chronic dehydration. By drinking more liquids they can reduce the frequency of attacks. They may even be able to control their condition completely just by drinking more. The prescription is simple: Drink eight fluid ounces, preferably water, every waking hour, starting in the morning upon arising.

For busy people on the move, carry a water bottle. Fluid is the key to controlling asthma. Fluids do not mean soda pop. Fizzy drinks should be avoided. The carbonation causes the diaphragm to rise and puts unwanted pressure against the lungs.

Many asthmatics are sensitive to substances in their surroundings. Such environmental offenders can trigger reactions, increase inflammation, and aggravate the asthmatic condition. If you or a child in your family are asthmatic, here are some ways to reduce your exposures:

- Encase bedding in allergen-impermeable covers to avoid contact with dust mites
- Wash sheets and blankets in hot water
- Exterminate cockroaches
- Avoid tobacco smoke
- Remove household pets from living quarters
- Decrease indoor humidity in order to minimize the presence of mold

Chapter Eighteen

Sinusitis

MSM has huge potential as a natural remedy for relief of the typical pain and discomfort of sinusitis, a problem suffered by many millions of people. More than two hundred patients at the Portland clinic have used it to date. Often MSM brings relief within a week or two, sometimes even faster. In about half of the cases, patients have told us that their sinus problem hasn't returned.

One such case involved Nic Wickliff, 64, a freelance Portland photographer who has been treated since 1972 for a severe back injury. During the 1980s, he developed a recurrent sinus infection with the typical pain, pressure, and thick mucus. Prescription medicines did not help him.

When Wickliff mentioned his stubborn problem during an office visit, it was suggested that he try a dilution of MSM crystals in water and apply the solution directly into his nose with a medicine dropper.

"I put a few drops into each nose a couple of times a day and the problem gradually cleared up within a couple of weeks," says

Wickliff. "I used the drops off and on for about six months and then stopped. The problem never returned."

Sinusitis is an inflammation of the tiny cavities close to your nose and eyes. Normally, air passes in and out of these spaces and is cleaned and filtered in the process. However, colds and allergies can cause swelling inside the cavities, resulting in infections and inflamation. Typical symptoms are headache, pressure around the face and eyes, thick mucus, and a persistent cold. Sinus infections can last for many weeks and become a recurrent problem.

Many chronic cases of sinus infections are allergic in nature. Food, dust, molds, pollen, and chemicals can inflame the sinus tissue.

Standard treatment of sinusitis includes antibiotics, decongestants, and steam to loosen mucus.

For relief with MSM, take the supplement orally on a daily basis but also administer it directly into your nose. Here's how to do it:

- Use an empty medicine dropper bottle or a small nasal-spray bottle. Patients tend to prefer the spray.

- Purchase a container of pure MSM crystals. Be sure the product does not contain other ingredients beside MSM.

- Depending on the size of the bottle, add slightly less than a level teaspoon of MSM crystals for each ounce of water. This quantity provides an optimum ratio of 15 percent MSM. If the mixture is a bit cloudy, it means that not all the MSM has gone into solution. MSM will dissolve more readily in warmer water. If you use more than this amount of MSM, some of the crystals will not dissolve.

- With a spray bottle, spray three or four times into each nostril several times a day.

- If you use a medicine dropper, fill it to a comfortable level and apply into each nostril several times a day.

- The MSM may cause a slight burning sensation. Most people say that after a day or two they get accustomed to it and then have no problem.

- Use this procedure as often as necessary.

Chapter Nineteen

Food Allergies

About Food Allergies

Classical allergies, such as a sensitivity to a pollen or a cat, show up immediately. You start sneezing or coughing on exposure. Food allergies, which are the result of a particular food or ingredient causing an irritation or inflammation of tissues in the body, are more tricky and challenging. Specialists say most food allergies or sensitivities, rather than causing sudden reactions, cause delayed reactions that may take anywhere from three hours to three days to be evident. This makes it harder to connect reactions to specific foods. Symptoms vary, ranging from GI tract disturbances, hives, and headaches, to behavioral changes.

Environmental-illness expert Doris Rapp, M.D., author of *Is This Your Child's World?*, reports that "repeated scientific studies have indicated that as many as 66 percent of children diagnosed with attention-deficit hyperactivity disorder (ADHD) actually have an unrecognized food allergy causing their symptoms."

Each of us have unique physiological and biochemical weak points, levels of immunity, and susceptibilities to illness, based on genetics. These, as well as the quality of diet and the amount of stress in our lives, also play a role in where, when, and how intense, allergic reactions develop.

MSM and Food Allergies

At the DMSO Clinic in Portland, many patients treated for interstitial cystitis, an inflammatory condition of the bladder, have mentioned that their food allergies have diminished after they started taking MSM. These are individuals with intolerances to many different foods. Commonly, an individual is allergic to more than just one food. The usual way of avoiding problems is to avoid the particular foods that offend.

MSM doesn't cure food allergies. However, patients say that in many instances MSM gives them tolerance to a food they could otherwise not eat. All that's needed apparently is to take MSM prior to, or during a meal, that contains the forbidden food.

Several patients have mentioned sensitivity to tomato sauce. They say that if they sprinkle MSM crystals on spaghetti topped with tomato sauce they have no problem. I have heard the same thing from people with allergies to citrus and certain vegetables. If they take MSM before they eat, they have no problem.

One MSM user wrote to say that she has food allergies and starts to sneeze and develop congesion whenever she eats more than one allergy-inducing food over a period of several days. "After two months on MSM I have had no symptoms from eating these foods," she said.

This interesting feedback has been volunteered by patients. It suggests that health professionals who focus on food sensitivities in their practice consider the use of MSM as a therapeutic tool.

One such physician is gastroenterologist Trent Nichols, M.D., medical director of the Center for Nutrition and Digestive Disorders in Hanover, Pennsylvania. He has found MSM helpful against food allergies, including his own.

"I used to take Imitrex (sumatriptan), a prescription medication, once or twice a week for migraines stemming from multiple food allergies," he says. "If I were to eat chocolate, for instance, I would normally have a migraine the next day. This situation has become worse over the last ten years despite all the remedies I have at my disposal.

"For myself, and for many of my patients who have not been able to get significant help for their food-allergy problems, MSM has made a huge difference. After starting on MSM, many of them are able to tolerate foods they couldn't handle before. They tell me they can now eat previously forbidden food without suffering from discomfort and adverse reactions afterward."

To date, about forty people in his practice with food allergies have said they benefitted from MSM since Nichols introduced it in 1997.

"These are patients already on a variety of programs and nutritional aids," he points out. "But when we added MSM they told us there was a noticeable improvement in well-being and tolerance to food.

"Relief among them has varied. It's always an individual thing. But they generally report a lessening of such gut-induced symptoms as bloat, distention, gas, constipation, and diarrhea. For some, the improvements have been dramatic. My clinic specializes in digestive disorders, so we look for these things.

"But people also tell us that their skin conditions improve. Or that their hives are less. Or their asthma improves. These include individuals taking steroids for hives or asthma. Often they can reduce their medication or stop taking it altogether."

Nichols says the improvements he observes usually start within a week.

"MSM may be helping to repair cell membranes in the gut," he suggests. "But perhaps the major thing is that is stabilizes the mast cells. I think that is really what is going on. It stabilizes these cells so that they don't produce as much histamine."

After starting on MSM some patients may develop a headache before they start to improve. "Patients have mentioned the headache," he says. "So I tell people to watch for it and if it does occur to drink a lot of water. This may possibly be some kind of a purification or detoxification effect being stirred up in the body by the MSM."

MSM is "an important piece of the puzzle, as important as anything we have been using and maybe more," says Nichols of the role of MSM in his nutritionally oriented practice. "I feel that MSM holds much potential and I would now like to do a study to verify the subjective and observational evidence."

Nichols recommends up to a teaspoon of MSM crystals twice a day to his patients.

"This level seems to work well," he says.

Part **FOUR**

How **MSM**

Helps Relieve

Other Pain

Problems

Chapter Twenty

Rheumatoid Arthritis, Lupus, Interstitial Cystitis, Scleroderma

A Mother's Story

Kristin Miller has been to hell and back even though she is only six years old. The journey, as her mother tells it, began with a backyard fall in 1994 at the Miller home in Fredericksburg, Virginia. Kristin was not quite two at the time.

"Her right knee became red, hot, and swollen," Dorothy Miller recalls. "The pediatrician called it a sprain and said to ice it and try to have her stay off the leg as much as possible. It would heal in a few weeks. Oh, how I only wish the doctor had been right.

"Kristin was happy, outgoing and adventuresome. After her fall, she was not her usual self. She became irritable, lost her appetite, and cried a lot, keeping us up at night. It became obvious after a short period of time that it was more than just a sprained knee. Tests determined she had a very aggressive form of juvenile rheumatoid arthritis.

"Then began a merry-go-round of medication, including

Advil, Naprosyn, and Children's Motrin. They didn't help much. She was crying all the time. Kristin's right knee became swollen to double the size of her left knee. It was a constant source of pain. She would contort the leg into unnatural positions in an attempt to ease the pain. Whatever position the leg was in when she fell asleep was the position it would be in the morning. It would be locked stiff and she would often be in pain and crying. I would put Kristin into a warm bathtub and have to manipulate her leg for an hour or two to loosen the contracture. She would crawl for a few hours afterward and then walk with a limp afterward. We eventually had to use a specially designed leg brace to keep her leg straight. Then her right ankle became swollen to the point that she couldn't wear a shoe on the foot.

"The doctors said she needed stronger medication and prescribed a steroid drug, Prelone. She took a high dose orally and it helped some with the swelling. But they don't like to keep children on steroids for any length of time because of side effects and potential damage to the body. The plan was to get relief from the steroids and then rotate to the nonsteroidal anti-inflammatories. Trouble was, the nonsteroidals didn't work and so she was kept on the steroids. The side effects were a nightmare, as bad as the disease itself. Kristin developed body hair and premature breast tissue, mood swings, demineralization in her bones, and a hunch in her back. Her immune system was shattered. Any minor cold became a crisis. For that reason she had to be isolated from other kids.

"She swelled up like a balloon. Her muscles were so weak she could hardly walk. She often had stomach pain and cried from the discomfort. Once she had constipation for many days and then suddenly, while standing, literally exploded with black, gritty feces. She was so toxic from the drugs. In 1995, the doctors said that the steroid medication should be reduced and eventually discontinued. They were concerned about Cushing's disease, a condition brought about by long-term drug treatment that affects the adrenal glands and results in the glands stopping the production of cortisol. Eventually, she was diagnosed with Cushing's.

"We were then given two choices for continuing treatment:

methotrexate, a chemotherapy drug, or gold shots. The options were like going from the frying pan into the fire. The risks included hair loss, vomiting, diarrhea, and liver damage for the methotrexate and excruciating pain with the gold shots. Even with these options, one doctor told me, the prognosis was very poor for Kristin.

"By this time I had lost faith in the doctors and started to search for other options on my own. I learned in my inquiries that methotrexate actually causes lymphoma in some children but it is said to clear up when the medication is stopped. Nevertheless, that kind of news was all I needed to hear. These aren't acceptable treatments. I also learned that the methotrexate is not even approved by the FDA for children, yet it is still used. I wasn't going to let my daughter be destroyed by torturous treatments.

"Early in 1996 I heard about the work of Dr. Jacob at the Oregon Health Sciences University. I contacted him and he suggested we try MSM. I told my pediatrician about it, who replied that it probably wouldn't harm—or help—my daughter. So we started her on MSM with orange or apple juice every day and also applied MSM lotion to her swollen joints.

"Within two weeks I started seeing changes. The pain was still there. But her appetite was better. Her disposition improved. She started laughing. I was afraid to believe what I was seeing. As time passed, there were more improvements. Her knee was less swollen. We slowly weaned her off the steroids and stopped the drug altogether by August 1996. By then, Kristin no longer needed the leg brace. She was walking better than ever, and the knee inflammation had subsided in a major way. The doctors said she was in remission. Could it be? I stopped the MSM and the symptoms started getting worse again. So I knew it was the work of MSM and not a true remission.

"By September 1997 Kristin was able to attend kindergarten. She was walking, running, full of energy, and seemingly less bothered by colds than other kids. She soon was able to become a Brownie and enjoy the fun activities like other girls her age.

"Kristin keeps taking her MSM regularly. I don't know where she would be without it. If not dead, then for sure in a lot of misery. She has some residual problems from her ordeal, but basically she is intact and healthy, with a chance for a normal, happy and pain-free life. That is all a mother can ask for."

About Rheumatoid Arthritis

Rheumatoid arthritis is a crippler, the most inflammatory of arthritic conditions. Unlike common wear-and-tear degenerative arthritis associated with aging, rheumatoid can strike at any age. It tends to affect more women than men, especially those between the ages of twenty and forty. Most often rheumatoid involves the extremity joints—the elbows, wrists, knees, feet, and hands. It is sometimes associated with low-grade fever and fatigue.

According to The Arthritis Foundation, more than 2 million people suffer with this condition in the U.S. Typically, rheumatoid tends to persist over prolonged periods of time. Joints become warm, swollen, tender, often red, and painful or difficult to move. If inflammation persists or is not responsive to treatment, destruction of adjacent cartilage, bone, tendons, and ligaments can develop, leading to deformity and disability. The Arthritis Foundation says that susceptibility or a tendency to develop rheumatoid can be inherited, but not everyone who inherits the susceptibility will develop the disease.

Rheumatoid arthritis is considered an auto-immune disease, meaning that a person's immune system starts attacking body tissue. Scientists don't know exactly why this happens. The interaction of multiple factors are involved in most cases. Hormonal changes or infectious agents may trigger the disease process in susceptible individuals. Nutritional deficiencies and food allergies are thought by many experts to contribute to the illness. Some studies have demonstrated that symptoms improve in many patients with the elimination of food allergies. In Kristin's case, her mother determined that her daughter was sensitive to soy, bananas, and dairy products. Prior to developing rheumatoid, the girl developed many ear infections, which Dorothy Miller thinks were related to a milk allergy. By observing her daughter's reactions, and through her own self-education, Miller was able to link offending foods to constipation, rashes, and aggravation of disease symptoms.

The standard medical approach has a dismal record for effectiveness and safety. The focus is mainly on suppressing symptoms. In the process, suffering patients frequently become casualties of the treatments themselves. Such treatments involve a three-stage approach, starting with aspirin, and then advancing to NSAIDs (nonsteroidal anti-inflammatory drugs) and steroids (cortisone), and finally chemotherapeutic agents.

NSAIDs, as we have mentioned earlier, generate serious side effects. One-quarter of the patients who take them develop ulcers within weeks. NSAIDs cause thousands of hospitalizations and 2,600 deaths annually in the treatment of rheumatoid arthritis alone. When NSAIDs fail, as they often do, physicians resort to steroid medication, which presents a major problem if used for any length of time because of the high risk of multiple and serious side effects.

Immune-suppressant agents, such as Imuran, and methotrexate, a chemotherapeutic drug used for cancer, are extensively used for rheumatoid patients. While these drugs may reduce symptoms, over time they may have devastating effects. A study published in the leading British medical journal *Lancet* in 1989 said that this type of drug strategy can increase the rate of disability and shorten lifespan when used long-term.

Stanley Jacob, M.D., Comments:

There is no cure for rheumatoid arthritis and a few capsules or teaspoons of MSM are not going to rid the body of this disease process. But MSM does offer potentially powerful relief. It can make life much more bearable as long as you continue to take it. A very large percentage of people with rheumatoid, both adults and youngsters, benefit from supplementation. In many cases, improvement is felt within a few days, making MSM a potent and attractive palliative option.

Many individuals report dramatic results. People have told me they started MSM after their rheumatologists could no longer help them and then returned months later to their surprised physicians appearing rejuvenated and virtually symptom-free.

The most severe case I personally treated involved a lawyer in his late fifties with advanced disease in his shoulders, knees, and hips. When I saw him he already had two knee replacements and would eventually need hip and shoulder replacements as well. His joints were in bad shape. He was taking very large doses of medication—3,200 milligrams of Motrin and 40 milligrams of Prednisone a day. Motrin is a nonsteroidal anti-inflammatory. Prednisone is a widely-used steroid medication often prescribed for rheumatoid. Both types of medications are medically important agents, however they are associated with serious side effects.

The lawyer said he knew I couldn't cure him, but he hoped I could give him better quality of life and enhance his ability to continue in his professional career. After a few months on MSM, he was greatly improved and down to 400 milligrams of Motrin and less than 5 milligrams of Prednisone. MSM often allows such a reduction in medication, even in severe cases, because of its pain- and inflammatory-relief properties. Sometimes MSM alone can control the condition so that no drugs are necessary, although in his severe case this wasn't possible. Today the lawyer maintains a busy practice. His pain is down 75 percent. He is not cured. But he is very happy.

At my Portland clinic, I have treated more than a dozen children—such as Kristin Miller—who have the severe juvenile form of the illness. More than two-thirds of them have been significantly improved. MSM has been effective in children as young as two and three years old. Parents report that their children, who are on high doses of risky medication, are often able to reduce and sometimes stop the prescription drugs after starting on MSM. This is good news because of the serious side effects of long-term drug use. Little Kristin was on huge doses of Prednisone but was not improving. Steroid therapy in youngsters can retard normal growth. That is what happened to Kristin.

Her reversal didn't happen overnight, but her inflamed joints are under control with MSM alone. Her laboratory tests are fairly normal now and she has no need for drugs, which would eat up her gastrointestinal tract. We believe her life has been changed without the threat of side effects looming over her.

An animal study by Jane Morton and R. D. Moore of the Oregon Health Sciences University in 1985 strongly suggested a healing role for MSM for this condition. The researchers used a particular strain of mice prone to the spontaneous development of joint disease similar to rheumatoid arthritis. Such animals have a lifespan of only five and a half months. For this experiment, the animals were divided into groups. Eighteen were given regular water to drink and fourteen drank water with 3 percent MSM. The trial began when the mice were two months of age and ended when they were four or five months old. At that time their knee joints were examined for degeneration of tissue.

Morton and Moore found that animals drinking regular water showed a breakdown in joint cartilage while those on MSM did not. Almost all of the control rodents had an inflammatory reaction developing in the synovial tissue (the lining of the joints), compared to half of the MSM mice. In the latter group, the degree of inflammation was less advanced. In addition to the "significant protection" from spontaneous development of rheumatoid joint disease, the researchers said that the MSM also reduced the amount of lymph-node disease and harmful autoimmune antibody activity normally associated with rheumatoid arthritis. They recommended more research to determine the precise mechanisms of MSM's anti-inflammatory and immune-modifying actions. I hope funding can be found for this purpose. The one promising animal study and the remarkable experience of many rheumatoid patients taking MSM clearly demonstrates a positive therapeutic role for MSM that merits scientific investigation.

Ronald Lawrence, M.D., Comments:

MSM offers major relief for rheumatoid arthritis. I have seen major improvement in as little as two days. Based on my clinical observation, glucosamine sulfate supplements, while useful for degenerative arthritis, have no effect on rheumatoid arthritis.

I recently treated a patient who told me about her seventy-eight-year-old mother who had been suffering many years with rheumatoid. I told her about the MSM and suggested she bring her mother in. The elderly woman was in great pain. She had deformed hands and walked, crouched over, with great difficulty. She had been on every possible medication during the previous twenty years. She couldn't tolerate some of the medication and had experienced many adverse side effects. I suggested trying MSM.

Four days later the older woman returned. She didn't have an appointment. She told my receptionist she just wanted to come and kiss my hand. When I saw her she was a new person.

"I can't believe what this powder has done for me," she said, beaming. "I can sleep again. For twenty years, sleep has been a problem because of the pain. Two nights ago, for the first time in years, I slept like a log. The pain started to go down soon after I began taking your powder. And it's been getting better every day. I just can't believe it."

Along with a gentle exercise program and the addition of important vitamins and minerals, this patient has continued to make a remarkable recovery.

Many of my rheumatoid patients report rapid and substantial relief from symptoms with MSM. Previously, if I was unable to help severe cases, I would refer them to a specialist. Now, I find this amazing supplement helps even the most severe conditions and gives me a substantial therapeutic tool. It doesn't restore destroyed joints but it makes the lives of patients much more comfortable and also produces many other side benefits.

Most of my patients have used cortisone or immune-suppressant drugs and had trouble with one or the other. Those are powerful agents with serious side effects. They should only be used as a last resort. The prospect of avoiding such drugs by using a simple supplement like MSM should make any physician and patient happy. It certainly did just that for actor James Coburn, who is one of my patients.

"Like a miracle":
James Coburn's Story

During the last half of his illustrious forty-year film career, actor James Coburn has been in pain every time he made a movie. The problem started in 1978, when his wrists became sore and swollen. The pain then began to affect other parts of his body.

"I was filming *Loving Couples* with Shirley MacLaine when one foot began to hurt, then the other, and then both legs, so that normal movement became very painful," Coburn recalls. "After filming ended I consulted with a doctor. Tests showed I had rheumatoid arthritis. The doctor said there wasn't much he could do. He gave me an anti-inflammatory prescription, which took a little of the edge off the pain, and told me to come back when I finished the prescription. I never went back."

The actor says that rheumatoid runs in his family. His father and an aunt had the disease. He believes that negative emotions associated with personal problems at the time triggered his illness.

The pain got so bad that Coburn couldn't perform for a time in major roles. "I was sick and in bed a lot of the time," he remembers. "Any movement was painful. I would break into a sweat just standing up. The pain was all over and constant."

Coburn set out on a personal health crusade to try to find—and correct—lifestyle, diet, and other controllable factors related to his illness. For more than fifteen years he tried fasting, colon cleansing, special food allergy elimination diets, deep tissue massage, acupuncture, electromagnetic energy, homeopathy, and even laying on of hands.

"The condition did get better with all the different things I tried but the pain and stiffness were always there and I still couldn't move very well," he says. "I could work but I was always in some pain.

"The condition also caused physical deformation. Tendons had become shortened. My arms were bowed. The fingers in the right hand were bent a bit. My left shoulder was always in pain. I tried to keep myself from deteriorating by doing some kind of a workout, either on a bicycle or light weights or walking, and just toughing out the pain. I felt that if I didn't I would just stiffen up. I felt I was healing myself slowly. But there was always pain. When it got too bad I would take aspirin."

In the beginning of 1998, Coburn was introduced to MSM. "It was like a miracle," he says. "The pain stopped. In three days I started to swing a golf club. I couldn't believe the difference."

After six months of MSM, the 70-year-old actor says he has virtually no pain at all and "sometimes zero." He takes a teaspoon and a half of MSM crystals twice a day mixed in hot water and adds juice. He is working with a personal trainer and has started to hit tennis balls in the hope that he can soon play tennis for the first time in twenty years.

"I can't tell you how good it feels," he says. "Psychologically, I feel like a human being again instead of a cripple struggling for some kind of freedom from pain."

Coburn says he still has bowed tendons and bent fingers. There is still stiffness but he keeps working it out. "Now if I have pain it is from stretching muscles and tendons beyond a range that they haven't been pushed to before. It is not the pain of arthritis," he says.

As far as his acting career is concerned, Coburn says that joy has returned to his work. After he started using MSM, he performed in a starring role as an alcoholic in *Affliction,* with Nick Nolte and Sissy Spacek.

"I play an old abusive father," says Coburn. "It was an active role and it was a lot of fun. I felt a new freedom. It was no longer painful to move. Before I couldn't move fast enough. I felt hesitant, out of synch, and out of rhythm. Lagging behind. I was always holding back, the fear of pain in the back of my mind. Curiously, I played in a movie called *Affliction,* and for the first time in years I didn't feel afflicted."

Lupus

"Is Mommy dead yet?":
Marian Gormley-Pekkola's Story

Shortly after delivering twin girls in 1985, Marian Gormley-Pekkola, of Carlton, Oregon, became severely ill—first with a strep infection and then severe rheumatic fever. Later she was diagnosed with lupus and myofibrositis, an inflammation of muscle tissue. The combination left her incapacitated, with systemic pain in the joints and muscles, drained of energy, and unable to care for her family. Her husband literally had to carry her from room to room in her house, and if he wasn't there, she crawled. For two years, a nanny cared for the children by day, while her husband took care of them at night.

Her two older boys, then aged seven and five, used to stand outside her bedroom door and talk about her condition in gloom-and-doom terms.

"Is mommy dead yet?" she heard them say on a number of occasions.

She was given antibiotics and extremely high doses of cortisone. She suffered side effects such as digestive upset and sleeplessness. Her physicians recommended narcotic analgesics for the constant pain, but she refused because she feared she would become dependent on the drugs. One of her doctors gave her less than a year to live.

"The average person might have waited to die, but I have always been a fighter," says Gormley-Pekkola. "I tried every possible treatment that was available, including laughter therapy and hypnotherapy, but nothing worked until I found MSM."

In 1987, a friend who had been treated at the DMSO Clinic in Portland told her about MSM and recommended that she make an appointment.

"Dr. Jacob suggested MSM and he gave me a supply of crystals, but frankly I had been through so many medical treatments that I was pretty skeptical," she says. "The container of crystals stayed unopened for two weeks or so before I got around to trying them. Finally I gave in and started taking them. I took a table-spoon three times a day. I didn't like the taste so I put the crystals in capsules."

According to Gormley-Pekkola, within ten days she experi-enced what she describes as a "miracle." The pain and fatigue started to lessen dramatically.

"Within a short period I was essentially free of the constant pain and fatigue," she says. "And I have remained that way ever since."

Today, Gormley-Pekkola is very much alive at the age of 46. She is a "fully-functioning Type-A person," as she says, an accoun-tant who manages three businesses with her husband. She walks up to five miles a day and is physically and emotionally very much involved in the activities of her four growing children.

Gormley-Pekkola says she takes the MSM on an as-needed basis. "If I have a flare-up with lupus or some related problem, I will take some of the crystals for a short period of time and that seems to resolve things. The MSM gave me back 95 percent of my health, and it's as if I was never ill. I have my life back, and it is a good life."

In so-called autoimmune diseases, the body's immune system becomes deranged or hyperstimulated and attacks its own tissue, causing pain, inflammation, and many symptoms. One such dis-order is systemic lupus erythematosus—or lupus for short—which can affect skin, joints, blood, and multiple organs.

According to the Lupus Foundation of America, lupus is more common than cerebral palsy, multiple sclerosis, sickle-cell ane-mia, and cystic fibrosis combined. One out of 185 Americans have lupus, among them ten to fifteen times more adult women than men. The exact cause is unknown, but evidence points to interre-lated immune, environmental, hormonal, and genetic factors. In an autoimmune condition, the body produces certain antibodies that target and destroy its own cells. In systemic lupus, these anti-bodies attack white and red blood cells, platelets, and cells of the joints, heart, kidneys, liver, blood vessels, and other organs. Joint pain and inflammation resembling rheumatoid arthritis is present in about 90 percent of patients. Sunlight provokes or may aggravate skin eruptions. Lymph nodes are typically enlarged.

MSM and Lupus

MSM can provide major relief for lupus. It can be used in conjunction with cortisone, the standard medication, or alone. By itself it improves joint, skin, and vascular symptoms. Patients taking MSM experience results at least as good as from taking cortisone, but without the side effects associated with the drug.

MSM doesn't cure lupus any more than cortisone does, but it is an effective treatment due in large part to its anti-inflammatory and immune-modulating actions.

Several dozen patients with lupus have been treated with overall good results. Almost three-quarters of them have benefited.

A promising role for MSM in auto-immune diseases was demonstrated by an animal study conducted at the Oregon Health Sciences University's Department of Arthritis and Rheumatic Diseases in 1986. The experiment involved mice prone to auto-immune proliferative diseases resembling leukemia and lymphoma in humans. Because of their susceptibility, the life span of these rodents is five and a half months. They develop anemia, lupuslike kidney disease, and enlargements of lymph nodes, spleen, and thymus.

In the study, one group of mice was provided either DMSO or MSM in their daily drinking water while the other group was maintained on normal water. After thirty-nine weeks, all of the nonsupplemented animals were dead. At forty-six weeks, nearly 80 percent of the supplemented mice were still living. On average, DMSO and MSM nearly doubled the lifespan of the animals to ten months.

The supplemented mice remained healthy and vigorous throughout their lives, observed researchers Jane Morton and Benjamin Siegel. The animals showed significant reduction of anemia and the typical enlargements of lymph nodes and spleen. Moreover, there were no signs of toxicity even on high doses of MSM— the equivalent of 6 to 8 grams per kilogram of body weight daily. By comparison, an adult human might take a *total* of 6 to 8 grams a day.

"We have found DMSO and $DMSO_2$ (MSM) to be virtually identical in their ability to diminish the severity of these disorders," Morton and Siegel reported in the journal *Proceedings of the Society for Experimental Biology and Medicine.* It is conceivable that $DMSO_2$, which is the major metabolite of DMSO in the body, "may be the biologically effective molecule in these reactions," they added. The precise mechanism for this protective role is yet unclear. The researchers suggested that MSM might alter the role of antibodies and other immune system elements as well as the activity of certain immune-regulating molecules such as prostaglandins.

In a follow-up study with laboratory rodents using the same model, DMSO and MSM were again found to extend life span as well as reduce the severity of anemia and kidney damage and lessen the degree of spleen enlargement. In this second study, some of the animals were started on DMSO and MSM when they were seven months old and their underlying terminal disease process was well underway. Even under these circumstances, their lives were extended substantially.

Morton and Siegel found a significant reduction in certain antibodies that react with DNA and cause kidney damage. "Although we are not sure about the mechanism of action, DMSO and MSM may act by decreasing inflammatory responses and the production of autoantibodies and immune complexes," they concluded, recommending further studies.

Systemic lupus in humans is a destructive disease. It typically damages kidneys, and many people with the condition require kidney transplants. When MSM is taken as a supplement, patients demonstrate improved kidney function.

It is interesting to note that in the animal studies the

researchers found that DMSO and MSM generated similar positive results. Since people generally won't take DMSO for a long period of time because of the odor, the potential use of MSM as a long-term adjunct to treatment is well worth exploring.

Interstitial Cystitis

Day and night pain:
Barbara Norman's Story

When it was bad, and it was bad often, elementary-school teacher Barbara Norman, 49, of Oakville, Ontario, would struggle through a morning at school and then have to turn her kids over to a substitute teacher for the afternoon.

"Day and night, the abdominal pain was bad, and the urgency was bad," she says. "It affected my sleep, my waking hours, every part of my life."

Norman started developing what her doctors felt were recurring urinary tract infections after the birth of her daughter in 1980. For years she was prescribed round after round of antibiotics.

"The symptoms would leave for a while and then return again—worse," she says.

At one point her physicians suggested cortisone for the urinary tract inflammation. Norman would have none of it. She had previously taken cortisone to control her asthma and stopped because of the side effects. In 1990, a urologist dilated the urethra and cauterized what he called "damaged tissue." Afterward, she had more pain.

A few years later she saw another urologist who recommended a new drug—Elmiron—which helped relieved her pain for several months but then lost its effectiveness. Moreover, it made her nauseous. In the beginning of 1998, Norman started taking MSM orally and by mid-year, when this book was being written, she was experiencing consistent relief without any side effects for the first time.

About Interstitial Cystitis

Imagine the pressure building up around your bladder to the point of pain and spasm so that you must desperately urinate thirty, forty, fifty, or more times a day. That's the ordeal faced by people such as Barbara Norman who have interstitial cystitis (IC). Your bladder is a balloon-shaped sac with elastic walls that expand to store urine. When you urinate, the walls relax. Inside the bladder, the connective tissue of the walls is protected from the waste products in the urine by a coating of mucous membranes. In IC, the membranes and underlying tissue become inflamed or irritated. Scarring, stiffening, and even bleeding develop in the tissue, along with a decreased bladder capacity.

Typically, there is an urgent need to urinate frequently both day and night. Pressure, pain, and tenderness in the pelvis and bladder area often increase as the bladder content rises and then decreases temporarily after it is emptied. The condition is believed to affect hundreds of thousands of people, most of them women in their twenties, thirties, and forties. Doctors don't know what causes it, nor do they have a cure. In the beginning, IC signs are similar to common cystitis, a urinary tract infection caused by bacteria and which responds to antibiotic treatment. However, IC is not caused by bacteria, and does not respond to antibiotics. Diagnosis is tough and doctors usually have to rule out other similar conditions. According to experts, thousands of cases are misdiagnosed, resulting in patients receiving treatments for which they experience only limited relief.

In the United States, interstitial cystitis is the only condition for which DMSO has been approved by the FDA as a prescriptive agent. We started using it in 1962 and today it is the medicine most widely used by urologists for IC. DMSO is applied intravesically, that is, as a kind of bladder wash. During weekly or biweekly treatments, the DMSO is instilled into the patient's bladder through a catheter and held for about fifteen minutes. Treatment cycles last up to eight weeks and then are repeated as necessary. Some patients are taught to self-instill. According to medical reports, patients who respond to DMSO usually experience improvements within about four weeks.

Stanley Jacob, M.D., Comments:

I have treated hundreds of moderate to severe IC patients for more than thirty-five years and 90 percent of them have experienced less pain, frequency, and urgency.

MSM may even be better than DMSO for this condition. DMSO stings as it enters into the bladder. MSM does not. This allows the patient to hold the solution longer in the bladder and therefore gain more benefit. Moreover, MSM doesn't produce the typical odor that discourages many people from continuing with DMSO.

Some years ago, after personally using MSM successfully for IC instillations in my clinic, I asked a leading expert on IC to test it—Stacy J. Childs, M.D., then at the University of Alabama-Tuscaloosa, and now in private practice in Cheyenne, Wyoming. Childs found the MSM instillations beneficial for several typical IC patients who had not been helped by other standard medications. The symptoms of each patient ceased after varying periods of treatment but then returned again some time after the experimental MSM solution ran out.

Although his study was small and not conducted in a tightly controlled manner, Childs was impressed enough to report his findings in a 1994 issue of the medical journal *Urologic Clinics of North America.* In his report, he concluded that the MSM "did as good a job as DMSO but without the side effect" of the unpleasant taste.

Childs concluded that the use of MSM as a bladder instillation should be evaluated in controlled studies. Such research, unfortunately, has not been done because of lack of funding. If conducted, I believe it will prove that MSM, without the odor and the occasional irritation, is superior to DMSO in the treatment of this condition.

Some patients have so much bladder inflammation that they cannot use the instillation method. Such patients are sometimes, but not always, able to control their symptoms on high doses of oral MSM (twenty to forty grams a day). Barbara Norman is an example. She experienced significant relief with supplementation alone.

Usually I find that IC patients don't have just bladder or urinary symptoms alone, but instead suffer multiple problems throughout the body, such as musculo-skeletal disability, intestinal irregularities, depression, and overwhelming fatigue. I have concluded that IC is not an illness localized in the bladder but rather is part of a systemic disorder.

Barbara Norman often felt fatigued, depressed, and sick, as if she had a "flu." "It wasn't just an isolated pain that you could try to ignore and life goes on around it," she says. "It involved my whole body."

Norman also suffered for many years from severe asthma and was told by doctors that it would shorten her life. The MSM not only relieved her IC symptoms, but she no longer wakes up at night because of breathing difficulty. She requires much less use of her inhalers. She says she has much more energy now and the constant unwellness she felt before has been replaced with a feeling of general wellness.

"It seems that such a large part of my life has been spent visiting doctors (both traditional and alternative) in an attempt to find relief for my illnesses," she says. "My health now is better than it has been for almost twenty years. I'm slowly getting back to full-time teaching again."

Localized bladder symptoms may be relieved when a urologist instills the bladder. The addition of a simple nutritional supplement like MSM offers relief for some of the systemic symptoms. In my experience, this combination approach yields the best results.

Scleroderma

The Joy of Wrinkles:
One Woman's Perspective

It's hard to imagine a woman being happy to see wrinkles on her face. Yet, in December 1986, Cindy Honaker of Norton, Ohio, was thrilled beyond words.

Shortly after she graduated from university thirteen years before and embarked on a teaching career, Honaker developed scleroderma, an extremely painful and crippling disease of the body's connective tissue. Skin turns rock hard and in its most destructive phase, the disease envelops the internal organs—the heart, lungs, kidneys, muscles, joints, blood vessels, and digestive tract—in a progressively tightening grip of scar tissue. The term scleroderma means scarred or hardened skin.

In 1986, Honakers's face was so tight that it had no wrinkles.

"When you smile, or when you furrow your brow, you get all those wrinkles, but I didn't have them," she recalls. "I had been doing twenty different facial exercises to get my face to loosen up. That's how desperate I was."

A friend with the same illness told Honaker about a lotion made from MSM.

"I applied it to my face and within two weeks my skin had softened to the point where I had wrinkles again." She laughs when she tells the story. "Not wrinkles of old age, or permanent wrinkles, but just the normal wrinkles you see when you make any normal facial expression. In the mirror, I lifted my eyebrows and there were wrinkles forming on my forehead. And when I relaxed my eyebrows, the wrinkles went away. It may sound strange that something like that could make you happy, but for me it was a miracle and the first sign of hope I had ever had with my disease."

Scleroderma usually begins with spasms of the small arteries throughout the body, often noticeable first in the fingers. As the condition progresses, the skin tightens, blood flow is impaired and ulcers develop at the fingertips, elbows, or ankles. Normal soft, supple skin becomes painful and calcified. The forearm and face become affected, while inside the creeping calcification spreads and interferes with the normal function of the body.

One year into her teaching career, Honaker had to stop working because the disease had taken over and no doctor or specialists could help her. "My body began to feel tighter and tighter, harder and harder," says Honaker. "It was very painful."

The fundamental cause of scleroderma is unknown. The condition has been linked to genetic predisposition, stress factors, and exposure to toxic substances, but research is minimal. In its worse form, the disease kills. Seven out of ten patients with severe scleroderma die within seven years of diagnosis. According to the Scleroderma International Foundation in New Castle, Pennsylvania, "Although some progress has been made in treating various symptoms, no effective treatment or cure for the overall disease has been discovered." The current estimate is that there are 500,000 to 700,000 people in the United States with scleroderma and 3,000 to 4,000 new patients per year. The condition most frequently starts between the ages of twenty-five and fifty-five and women are two or three times more likely to develop scleroderma than men.

Outside of the United States, DMSO is widely used for this condition. In Russia, for instance, it is the treatment of choice and often referred to there as the "cure" for scleroderma. We don't talk in terms of cure, but rather that it works well where doctors are willing to use it and know how to use it. Experts have urged that DMSO be approved as a prescriptive medication for scleroderma in the U.S.; however, such approval has never been granted.

Stanley Jacob, M.D., Comments:

For twenty-five years I have been medical director of the Scleroderma International Foundation. At my Portland clinic, I have treated hundreds of patients who have come from great distances. These are often end-of-the-line cases, patients taking penicillamine, steroids, anti-depressants, cortisone, methotrexate (a cancer drug), and immuno-suppressants, and they still are getting nowhere.

Many times, in addition to the symptoms of the disease, patients develop severe side effects from multiple drugs. Some on high doses of cortisone develop high blood pressure, psychoses, and humps in the back.

Patients often develop severe scarring of the esophagus. They cannot swallow well. Solid food becomes lodged in the esophagus. They frequently lose their appetite. They drop in weight and suffer from lack of energy. Metal tubes sometimes have to be surgically inserted to dilate the esophagus gradually so patients can swallow. An over-production of gastric acid may creep up into the esophagus to compound the destructive process of the disease itself. In Cindy Honaker's case, her gastroenterologist said her esophagus was "almost solid like a lead pipe." It had a diameter the size of a pencil. In an age before effective acid blocking medications, the acid had eaten away the valve at the lower end that opens into the stomach. For eleven years, she underwent esophageal dilations. She weighed eighty-two pounds as a result of not being able to eat normally.

Years ago, I treated this condition with DMSO and had excellent results. Then, as I began using MSM, I found that the results were even better. Because of the odor associated with DMSO, people often will not continue to take it indefinitely. MSM has no odor. Patients are thus more inclined to continue using it.

We know that many of the benefits of DMSO are due to the action of MSM. MSM performs major repair work in the body. It increases blood supply, which helps the healing process, and it functions as an analgesic and anti-inflammatory. Moreover, MSM softens scar tissue. In the esophagus, this effect results in an increase of the functional diameter of the tube. Patients then have more food choices and can eat more solids. Appetite, weight, and energy increase. This is what happened to Cindy Honaker. She was able to eat normally again.

Patients as severely affected as Honaker require intravenous treatment and then usually continue on oral and topical MSM. I recommend MSM both orally and topically. In serious cases, very large doses are necessary. The best results are usually seen in early cases. Nevertheless, even people with advanced disease may experience some degree of improvement. About 70 percent of scleroderma patients on MSM experience some degree of improvement. Under the supervision of regular physicians, they are frequently able to reduce their routine medication, which means they may have fewer side effects with which to contend.

MSM does not cure scleroderma. Patients must keep taking it. In general, it works gradually. There are no overnight miracles for this terrible disease. Patients begin to see a little softening of the skin. Hair that has been lost on the arms and legs starts to grow back. Typically, it takes a couple of months before patients notice significant improvement. But they usually do see results. At the worst, it will do nothing. At the best, it will help bring the condition under better control and heal painful ulcers.

As someone who has treated scleroderma patients for many years, I have seen MSM make a huge difference in many cases. I don't think it puts people into remission, but it has the potential to allow patients to function at a more productive and comfortable level in life, and with less pain.

Medical research is investigating why the body goes out of control in this terrible way. Until the answers and a better treatment are available, I urge all my scleroderma patients to take MSM.

If Vincenza Puccio had waited for medical science to come up with the answers she would have been dead long ago. Thirty years ago, scleroderma began developing in her hands. The skin became taut, her fingers stiff and painful. The tightness spread to her face, pulled at the skin around her eyes, giving her an almost Oriental appearance. The tightness then spread to her feet and elsewhere on her body.

"It was as if my body was slowly and painfully turning to stone," she remembers.

After rounds of medical tests and consultations, a specialist finally diagnosed her with scleroderma and said her condition was so aggressive that she probably wouldn't live for more than a year. Puccio's hands had hardened and become almost clawlike. She couldn't turn the ignition key in her car. She couldn't manipulate door knobs. She couldn't change her grandson's diapers. There were many times when she would cry out in pain just from the slightest movement. Often, husband Nick, a retired Army officer, would have to help her out of bed.

But Puccio shattered her doctor's bleak prediction. Today, she is very much alive. In fact, she is very active and owns and operates "2001 Cuts," a hair salon in Burke, Virginia. Her condition is well under control. Initially, she was treated with DMSO but for the last ten years she has maintained herself with an MSM supplement and gel.

She takes two and half tablespoons of MSM morning and evening and at the end of the day faithfully rubs down her tired and sore hands with an MSM gel.

"If I didn't do it, I couldn't work. My hands would tighten up and stiffen. I wouldn't even be able to hold a blow dryer," she says. "Today, I'm basically fine. I work. I do everything. I have no pain. My hands are still a bit firm, but they were like claws before. I know I wouldn't be here if it weren't for the MSM."

Cindy Honaker's life also took a positive turn with MSM. "There were no instant changes," she recalls. "Things just kept getting gradually better. Month after month, there was less and less pain. I had skin ulcers on my elbow that did not heal in fourteen years. There was nothing any doctor gave me that would help. I sometimes would walk the floor at night because of the pain from the ulcers. The ulcers also healed with MSM and never returned. Since 1987, I have never had to have my esophagus dilated again."

Honaker, now 47, was never able to return to the teaching career abbreviated by her illness. The condition weakened her immune system to the extent that she is ultra-susceptible to germs. Nevertheless, she shops, hikes, helps her widowed mother at home, eats "everything except spicy foods," and is relatively pain-free. She started the first chapter of a scleroderma self-help organization in Ohio and volunteers her time to the Arthritis Foundation and causes for the disabled.

Every day, Honaker looks in the mirror not the way most women do. She checks for wrinkles in a very special "scleroderma way." As long as they are there, she knows she is OK.

Appendix A

EXTRA BENEFITS

In addition to pain and allergy relief, people taking MSM supplements frequently experience these other benefits:

- relief of constipation
- lessening of scar tissue
- softer skin, thicker hair, and less brittle nails
- more energy

MSM and Constipation

Colon disorders read like a who's who of wretchedness—from bloating and abdominal pain to diverticulitis, inflammatory bowel conditions, and colon cancer. Constipation is right up there at the top of the list—a condition in which bowel movements are infrequent or difficult. Waste products stay longer in the system and become smaller and harder to expel. In time, the colon becomes a waste dump for toxins, bacteria, and carcinogens, a breeding ground for disease and malfunction.

Constipation can usually be "cured" by eating enough fiber in your diet, drinking enough water, and getting adequate exercise. For people doing all these good things for colon health and who still have a constipation problem, MSM is an ideal remedy.

Stanley Jacob, M.D., Comments:

As a dietary supplement, MSM offers great potential for anyone with constipation. MSM produces a general "tonic" effect in the bowels and normalizes bowel function, particularly for older individuals. We have given MSM to nursing homes, where constipation is a common problem. The nurses have said that MSM works well for patients, even for individuals not responding to Metamucil or stool softeners.

Patients being treated for arthritis or other painful conditions often say that MSM has restored their normal bowel movement. One patient recently said, "I now have normal bowel movements similar to when I was younger." One woman who started taking MSM said that within three days she had a "massive evacuation" and has been having a solid bowel movement every day since "which has never been the case with me."

A few elderly patients have obtained relief from constipation with very small doses of MSM, as little as 100 milligrams. In many cases, more may be needed—between a half-gram (500 milligrams) and 5 grams a day.

The use of sulfur in large doses as a laxative dates back to antiquity. Sulfur and molasses, a folk remedy from yesteryear, was given for a laxative effect. The sulfur in MSM may provide that same benefit.

Relief from constipation may also stem from MSM's ability to inhibit cholinesterase, an enzyme that slows down or blocks the flow of impulses along nerve pathways. As people get older, damage or increased inefficiency in the nervous system results in cholinesterase having a more pronounced role in slowing down impulses to the gastrointestinal tract. Constipation is common to many conditions related to the aging process. Nerve damage associated with diabetes, for instance, can slow normal bowel transit. Think of the intestines as a big muscle. It contracts and dilates to move food waste through the bowels and out of the body. If it weren't for cholinesterase, the intestines would go wild. But now, with age, and decreased efficiency in the nervous system, cholinesterase slows down the peristalsis too much. We develop sluggish bowels and constipation.

If you inhibit the action of cholinesterase you restore the ability of the nerve impulses to flow more smoothly and reach their intestinal muscle destinations. MSM inhibits the inhibitor, so to speak. It blocks the blocking action of cholinesterase.

One of the characteristics of MSM is that if you take too much of it, you can develop an increased stool frequency. In a sense, we use this effect to help people with constipation. For individuals with constipation, the result, however, is not diarrhea, but a normalcy of bowel movements. Our recommendation is to use the MSM as an aid to bowel normalcy by itself or use it along with whatever else you may be doing.

Ronald Lawrence, M.D., Comments:

Among my pain patients are individuals who also have chronic constipation or sluggish bowels. Many of them notice better bowel movement, and, as a result a feeling of greater well-being, after they start MSM. Now, when a patient mentions constipation, I have an extra reason to recommend MSM. Some patients are long-time users of laxatives. After patients use such medications for a long period of time, bowel function can deteriorate. But even for them, MSM is beneficial.

Promoting evacuation in this natural way is beneficial in a general sense. The faster you can move wastes and toxicity out of the body the better you feel and the less risk you have of developing serious colon disorders.

Caution: Any persistent change in bowel regularity should be checked by your physician. Although there tends to be a slowdown as part of the aging process, constipation could also be the sign of disease and a medical problem of concern.

Scar Tissue

Scar tissue formation is a normal aftermath of the body's response to injury. When you undergo an operation or sustain an injury, the natural intelligence of your body wants to reconnect or "knit" the damaged tissues, and scarring is the visible sign of the successful conclusion of this repair process. Unfortunately, the pieces don't usually heal up to their pre-damaged state.

If you are a runner, for instance, and undergo a knee operation, the scar tissue that forms never quite gives you the same knee you originally had. The knee may heal up 95 percent or more, but it's extremely rare that it returns to 100 percent. An operation is like an injury. You take a knife. You cut the skin. You cut the subcutaneous tissue. You bring about scar. We have never seen an incision heal without some scar.

If you were to line up a group of individuals with similar wounds who have undergone otherwise normal healing, you would see scarring but varying degrees of it. The reasons are not completely understood, but one appears to be due to a process in the collagen, the primary protein component in the healed wound, called "cross-linking." Abnormal increases in the cross-linking in collagen enlarges the bulk of a scar.

Scar tissue can cause residual stiffness and decreased range of motion. Frequently, pain develops at the site of a scar. This is due to small nerve fibers becoming "entrapped" and compressed in the scar tissue.

Over time, scar tissue diminishes. There tends to be a contraction as some normal adjacent tissue grows in. You will have a bigger scar two weeks after an abdominal operation than you will have six months later. But you won't ever be without a scar.

MSM and Scarring

MSM normalizes the cross-linking process. The was determined years ago in laboratory experiments. The practical effect of this is that when MSM is taken orally as a supplement and/or used as a gel or lotion topically it helps lessen scar formation and reduces the potential for pain. MSM does not eliminate scarring, but it helps, and even many years after the formation of a scar, it may alter scar tissue in a positive manner.

When MSM is taken before surgery, scars tend to be smaller. It may work as well as any agent currently available to minimize post-surgical adhesions and scarring. In this respect, MSM acts like DMSO, which is used topically by many plastic surgeons before and after procedures to minimize the amount of scar tissue.

For best results, start taking MSM before surgery and continue afterward. Once the dressing comes off and the wound is closed, apply topical MSM to the affected site.

MSM's ability to reduce scars occurs both externally and internally. In the case of chronic pulmonary disorders such as emphysema, asthma, and bronchitis, this property helps make the breathing process easier. MSM may also lessen the prominence of stretch marks. Start using it right after childbirth. The marks won't disappear, but you should start seeing a reduction within two months.

MSM and Keloids

Keloids are thick, protruding scars resulting from excessive amounts of collagen in healing tissue. They occur after surgery, burn wounds, and frequently after ear piercing, and develop more frequently on the upper part of the body, particularly the ear lobes, the borders of the jaw, the shoulder, and the chest. Thicker scars are associated with some types of cosmetic surgery, notably ear pinbacks, breast reductions, and tummy tucks.

MSM gradually softens and reduces such heavy scar tissue and makes it less prominent. If you put MSM to use for this purpose, be patient. The reduction process can takes months and even years, and will not completely remove the scar.

One of the most dramatic MSM stories involves Bill Rich, 64, a Portland mechanic and businessman. In 1970, he was trapped in a burning van for twenty minutes following a highway collision and was severely burned over a large area of his body.

"The fire cooked me on the right side from my knee up to the armpit," Rich says.

Extensive skin grafting left his body covered with scar tissue and adhesions, severely inhibiting normal activity. Even minimum physical effort was enough to stop him in his tracks, crying in pain. He was unable to walk more than a block a day.

"I had a patchwork of keloid scars like welding slag from the burns and skin grafts," he says. "One-third of me was twisted purple tissue. Frankenstein was good-looking by comparison. I measured the total length of all my scars once and they were sixty-five feet."

For seventeen years, Rich was often kept awake at night by the pain. In 1987, a veterinarian suggested he try a nutritional supplement used for pain in horses and other animals. The supplement was MSM. After three days, Rich says, most of the pain related to his scar tissues and adhesions was gone. As a sergeant in the Oregon State Defense Force, he was soon able to march with his troops.

Rich later made a lotion from the MSM and applied it regularly over the areas of his body that had been burned. With time, the knots of purple scarring—years old—started to shrink and were replaced by healthy pink skin. Today, he says, virtually all the scarring is gone.

MSM for the Skin, Hair, and Nails

One day in the summer of 1998, as we were writing the book, two women independently called the Portland clinic and excitedly remarked how their wrinkles had "vanished" after they started taking MSM. Does MSM really get rid of wrinkles? they wanted to know.

The answer is that MSM does a lot of good things for the body but there is no evidence that it erases wrinkles. Many women observe that it makes their skin softer. This effect probably also softens the wrinkle lines.

"Well, that's good enough for me," one of the callers said. "I'm happy with what I'm seeing. You should probably call MSM an internal cosmetic."

MSM is one-third sulfur, and sulfur has a reputation for being nature's "beauty mineral," for keeping the hair healthy and the complexion youthful. Skin, hair, and fingernails are normally quite high in cystine, one of the sulfur amino acids that gives keratin, a particular kind of protein found in these tissues, its property of toughness.

As physicians who treat patients for pain disorders, we are not experts in the field of cosmetics. But we do receive frequent feedback from our patients about how surprised they are to experience the cosmetic bonuses of MSM: softer skin, harder nails, and thicker hair. This gives us additional clinical evidence that MSM is a biologically active source of sulfur that is utilized by the body. We have it from long-time users that even in hot, skin-harsh places like Las Vegas, MSM keeps the skin soft and pliable. One such person is Sally Christy, 58, a contract administrator for a public utility in Nevada. She has been using an MSM lotion as a makeup base for more than twenty years.

"People tell me how soft my skin is, and for somebody my age living in a dry climate, where skin can easily become brittle, a natural product like this is a blessing for my skin," she says. "If you live out here in the desert for a long time, the climate starts to show on your face. My experience is that it definitely helps ward off wrinkling and keeps my skin youthful. I could buy any moisturizer on the market, but I don't need it. I choose to stick with MSM because it has worked so well for me."

Far from the sun and sand of Las Vegas, in Burlington, Ontario, Liz Miners of Lizanne's Hairdressing Salon has turned many of her clients on to MSM. Just as Christy does, Miners suggests the lotion as a makeup base.

"Cleanse your face as normal, then rub in some of the lotion. It helps the makeup go on smoother. You see softer, more pliable skin," she says. "Dry, scaly skin becomes more supple. Some people notice the change right away. For others, with bad skin conditions, it takes a while."

Miners recommends both the external lotion and the sulfur-rich MSM crystals to feed the skin from the inside. She uses the lotion twice a day and takes a teaspoon (about five grams) of crystals in an ounce of water once a day.

"You can use the lotion on your face, arms, feet, and hands," she states. "It has healing benefits wherever you put it. One of my customers is a woman with dermatitis. The face and neck would always look slightly scalded. She has been using cortisone creams for many years and they don't seem to be doing much for her anymore. She takes about five grams of the crystals every day with the lotion. After five weeks her skin has almost cleared up totally. She is pretty amazed. A friend used the lotion on her heels, which were always leathery and cracking. It was very uncomfortable for her. After three or four weeks her heels became much softer. She stopped using the MSM and the condition returned. Now she uses it continually and her heels are better again."

MSM speeds hair growth as well, says Miners. "That's good for my industry," she quips. "And the hair seems thicker. I do a lot of hair coloring and quite often when you color the hair you can take a hair strand and break it. The process may in some way weaken the hair. I've noticed that after people start taking MSM on a regular basis that their hair is stronger."

It's the same for nails. "They grow faster and stronger," she says. "Nails aren't as brittle. You don't seem to have as many hangnails."

Ronald Lawrence, M.D., Comments:

Stronger fingernails is a common "side effect" mentioned by female patients. These are often individuals with a lifelong history of fragile, brittle nails. After taking MSM regularly for a month or longer, they happily tell me their nails have become tough and no longer splitting or breaking off.

Recently I met a young woman in a neighborhood health food store whom I recognized as a check-out cashier in the supermarket where I often shop. We started chatting and she mentioned a problem with splitting nails. She was frustrated at her inability to grow long nails. I mentioned MSM to her and she said she would try it. I saw her again a couple of months later in the supermarket. She excitedly held her hands up. "Look," she said, "that stuff you told me to take really works!"

MSM for Energy

Haruo "Foozie" Fujisawa has been playing the drums professionally at clubs and private parties for more than a half century. The Los Angeles musician, now 76, limits his gigs to a few nights a week because, as he puts it, "drumming takes a lot out of you when you get to be my age."

Fujisawa started MSM early in 1998 and found that the supplement energized his drumming routines. "After a couple of weeks, I noticed much more stamina and energy," he says. "I do three or four solos a night and that takes strength and energy. Friends are now calling me a seventy-six-year-old marvel. I can beat the drums longer and harder."

Like Fujisawa, many patients report more energy after starting MSM. We don't know exactly what brings this about, but obviously people who are in less pain are going to feel better. But even healthy individuals and athletes have reported increased energy.

Some users of MSM are so delighted with the energy boost that they sit down and write us about it. Here are two samples of comments we have received:

● "I've had low energy all my life and I never realized how much I had slowed down until I started taking MSM. The first thing I noticed was more energy."

● "I'm a mountain biker and two or three times a week I take a pretty long and steep ride in the local mountains. My strength and endurance has improved. Somehow the MSM helps me utilize oxygen more effectively, resulting in less shortness of breath during the steeper more challenging climbs. Once I ran out of MSM and didn't take it for a week or two. I noticed almost immediately that uphill climbs that had become relatively easy were now difficult and required several stops to catch my breath."

TRUTH OR FICTION—SIFTING
THROUGH THE MSM CLAIMS

MSM has become a hot item at health food stores and drug stores. Some merchants display signs in their storefront windows declaring: "YES—WE HAVE MSM!" MSM is also being aggressively marketed by Internet and multi-level vendors.

Accompanying the growing interest in MSM and the marketing enthusiasm, a number of inaccuracies and erroneous claims have taken root and proliferated. The danger of such excess and distortion is to plant doubts about MSM's real value and give false hope to people suffering with very serious illnesses who should seek proper care. In this appendix, we are attempting to set the record straight. We have sifted through many of the widely circulated claims and assessed them according to current knowledge about MSM. We feel that consumers deserve the truth as best as we can determine it.

Claim: *"MSM is a free-radical scavenger (antioxidant)."*
Comment: A definitive determination as to whether MSM is

an antioxidant capable of substantial free-radical neutralization has not yet been made. Research has shown that DMSO is one of the most powerful antioxidants.

Claim: *"The body uses up one-eighth of a teaspoon of MSM each day during resting time alone."*
Comment: There are no data showing this.

Claim: *"Without the proper amount of MSM in our bodies, the amino acids will continue to build the glands, but fail to produce the correct enzymes, making us prone to unnecessary illness."*
Comment: There is no evidence for this.

Claim: *"If you drink rainwater you'll get the MSM, but if the city water supply adds chlorine, the MSM turns useless."*
Comment: The amount of MSM in rainwater is described as minuscule by atmospheric chemists. There is no evidence connecting MSM in rainwater to health benefits. Nor is there evidence that the city water supply has any effect on MSM.

Claim: *"MSM detoxifies the body."*
Comment: There is no scientific evidence for this. We have heard that some health professionals are using MSM for this reason but it needs to be investigated. DMSO has the chemical ability to bind with toxic metals and take them out of the body. MSM does not have this ability.

Claim: *"MSM is an anti-venom that can quickly bind up foreign proteins such as snakebites, flea bites, black widow bites, bee stings, and mosquito bites."*
Comment: Over the years, responsible individuals have told us how people and animals alike have been aided by MSM after snake and insect bites. It is an interesting use of MSM, but we have not personally had any experience with it. Some people have applied MSM crystals or lotions to multiple stings and said it reduced pain and inflammation. MSM may be help-

ful in such cases, but we have no concrete proof. The best response is to use well-established first-aid methods and seek medical help.

Claim: *"MSM makes cell walls permeable, allowing water and nutrients to freely flow into cells and allowing wastes and toxins to properly flow out."*
Comment: DMSO has this ability. It is an exciting property that implies an ability to facilitate the elimination of cellular toxins. MSM has not been studied for this effect and we are unsure if it has the same property. MSM itself passes through some cell membranes but there is no evidence that it renders the membrane more permeable to other compounds.

Claim: *"Without MSM, new cells in the body are not permeable, and osmosis is hampered."*
Comment: There is no evidence for this.

Claim: *"MSM opens the membrane in the brain that contains the aluminum and allows the unwanted deposits to be flushed into the bloodstream."*
Comment: There is no evidence to substantiate this.

Claim: *"MSM prevents over-reaction to other medicines."*
Comment: There is no basis for this claim. The use of MSM as a regular daily supplement has enabled many patients to reduce their medication. This is a result of MSM's ability to reduce pain and inflammation.

Claim: *"MSM controls acidity in the stomach, so it can help ulcers?"*
Comment: MSM will allow patients who have recurrent peptic ulcers to have fewer and less severe symptoms. Patients with heartburn experience less discomfort.

Claim: *"MSM coats the intestinal tract so parasites lose their ability to hang on. They are then flushed away."*

Comment: MSM has anti-parasitic properties but the precise modes of action have not been determined. We have no knowledge of MSM "coating" the intestines.

Claim: *"When you take MSM the pH in your body becomes normal."*
Comment: We are unaware of any evidence showing this.

Claim: *"When you take MSM your pH goes normal. Candida can not live in your body when your pH is normal—except in the colon where it belongs—so the Candida dies out. This is how MSM cures people of Candida. Just that simple."*
Comment: We have heard reports about MSM helping people with candida but we have not personally treated patients with this problem. We are unaware of any effect on pH.

Claim: *"MSM is no more toxic than water. It can never hurt anyone. If you overdose the extra MSM becomes inert and just passes through your system."*
Comment: MSM is very safe and indeed considered to be no more toxic than water. To date, there have not been any toxic effects or serious side effects associated with MSM. There is no evidence that if you "overdose" on MSM it becomes inert and just passes through the system. If you take too much, you may experience some minor GI discomfort or increase the peristalsis in your bowels and defecate more often as a result.

Claim: *"MSM is necessary for collagen synthesis."*
Comment: It plays a role in collagen synthesis. We don't know precisely yet how necessary it is or how big a role it has.

Claim: *"MSM reduces wrinkles."*
Comment: We would love to make this claim. Unfortunately, we can't. MSM, however, does make the skin softer and smoother.

Claim: *"MSM speeds healing."*
Comment: Clinical evidence indeed shows that MSM speeds healing of musculoskeletal injuries and inflammation.

Claim: *"MSM can change a cancer cell into a non-malignant cell."*
Comment: Several rat studies at Ohio State University and Oregon Health Sciences University have shown that MSM significantly slows the development of mammary and colon tumors when animals are given chemical substances that cause cancer. In these studies, MSM did not prevent the cancer, but delayed the disease in a major way. In the breast cancer study, for instance, MSM delayed the appearance of tumors by an average of one hundred days. Translated to human life, one hundred rodent days is the equivalent of about ten years. We need much more research to determine if MSM can slow the progress of cancer in humans. DMSO has the ability to change a cancer cell. The process is called maturation. It means that if you expose cancer cells to DMSO you alter them in a way. They look and act more like normal cells. In practical terms, this means that the use of DMSO allows you to reduce the dosage of a therapeutic agent, such as chemo. DMSO is in fact the most potent maturating agent known to chemistry, biology, and medicine. Many clinics in Europe and South America use it for this purpose. No such studies have been done with MSM.

Claim: *"MSM makes it possible for an alcoholic to come down off the alcohol without any of the withdrawal side effects."*
Comment: We have never observed this effect.

Claim: *"MSM relieves stress."*
Comment: Patients say they feel less depressed. MSM relieves pain and a person is likely to feel less stressed as a result. DMSO has been found useful in the treatment of psychoses. MSM has many of the properties of DMSO and it is possible that it could have an effect here as well. Research is needed.

Claim: *"MSM increases the ability to concentrate."*

Comment: Many people say this. MSM reduces pain. With less pain on one's mind, the ability to put attention on other matters would appear to be enhanced. This is an interesting connection that deserves to be investigated.

Claim: *"MSM increases the body's ability to produce insulin and is important for carbohydrate metabolism."*

Comment: MSM is helpful for diabetic neuropathy of the extremities and gastrointestinal tract. We have not seen MSM reduce the requirement for insulin or any anti-diabetic oral medication. It is an area that should be studied.

Claim: *"Diabetics who have been 'on the needle' for years can benefit from MSM supplementation. Some people are self-regulating since they discovered MSM."*

Comment: All diabetics should be under the care of a physician and modify their medication only on the basis of professional medical advice. If you are a diabetic, we invite you to show this book to your physician and ask if MSM would be appropriate for you.

Claim: *"Diverticulosis is an MSM and vitamin C deficiency."*

Comment: Diverticulosis is the most common disease of the colon and is typically caused by low-fiber diets. It is rare among individuals who routinely eat fiber-rich foods such as whole grains and vegetables. In diverticulosis, saclike pockets or herniations develop in the lining of the colon that become filled with fecal matter and toxins, causing swelling, inflammation, and pain. There is no evidence that this condition is related to an MSM or vitamin C deficiency, although both might help reduce some of the symptoms.

Claim: *"Vitamin C keeps MSM active in the system so you should take vitamin C with it."*

Comment Vitamin C is a wonderful substance. We know of

no evidence, however, for any specific supporting role related to MSM.

Claim: *"MSM deficiency aggravates many conditions."*
Comment: There is no known disease associated with a deficiency of MSM. People have not been measured for a deficiency of MSM. We have found clinically that many symptoms improve when MSM is used as a daily nutritional supplement.

Claim: *"MSM deficiency aggravates elevated cholesterol."*
Comment: There is no documented connection between MSM and cholesterol in humans. In laboratory experiments conducted by Don Layman of the Department of Anatomy at Louisiana State University, MSM was found to slow the degradation of low-density lipoproteins (the so-called "bad cholesterol") and spread of certain cells involved in blood vessel plaque. This research was conducted with cell cultures taken from bovine aortas. It is not possible to form an opinion about MSM's role against arterial disease based on such limited laboratory experimentation. Much more research is needed.

Claim: *"MSM deficiency aggravates migraine headaches. Supplementation can melt migraines away."*
Comment: There is no documented connection between MSM and migraines. MSM may help reduce the pain of headaches by relieving muscle spasm in the neck. In our experience we haven't found that it has an effect against migraines.

Claim: *"MSM deficiency aggravates Alzheimer's disease."*
Comment: There is no documented connection between MSM and Alzheimer's.

Claim: *"MSM deficiency aggravates rheumatoid arthritis."*
Comment: MSM, as a dietary supplement and a topical gel, helps rheumatoid arthritis patients because it relieves pain and

reduces inflammation. But deficiencies of MSM have not been measured in people.

Claim: *"It is the MSM in aloe vera leaves that soothes and repairs skin that has been cut, scraped, or damaged."*
Comment: There is no evidence for this. The MSM content in aloe vera leaves has never been measured as far as we know. There are sulfur compounds in aloe vera but we do not know if they include MSM.

Claim: *"A deficiency of MSM causes emphysema and supplementation of MSM can reverse it."*
Comment: MSM helps patients breathe easier. They don't get out of breath as easily. They can walk farther. It doesn't cure emphysema but it helps.

Claim: *"Women don't have the headaches, hot flashes, cramps, and nausea associated with the monthly cycle when they use MSM."*
Comment: The feedback is inconsistent, but some women have reported relief. This is probably due to MSM's ability to inhibit pain impulses and reduce inflammation.

Claim: *"MSM eliminates varicose veins."*
Comment: Typical varicose veins develop from pressure and weakness in the walls and valves of the veins in the legs—a mechanical problem. If the varicosity is associated with inflammation, as it sometimes is, the MSM will reduce the inflammation and may allow you to stand longer.

Claim: *"MSM takes out inflammation, permits the muscles to heal, and prevents them from becoming sore."*
Comment: Oral MSM reduces inflammation and muscle soreness. Reduction of pain follows. Topical application of MSM seems to further reduce muscle soreness. Using it topically also puts more MSM into the body, so there is an enhanced effect. Many athletes are using MSM to reduce the typical muscle soreness and inflammation that follow hard training sessions.

Claim: *"If you play sports or work out in a gym and normally get sore muscles the next day, take MSM before exercise and you will notice a difference. If taken after exercise, the soreness will go away faster."*

Comment: Many athletes and fitness enthusiasts are using MSM for this purpose. The supplement helps substantially in many cases.

Claim: *"MSM improves athletic performance."*

Comment: MSM won't help you run a three-minute mile but it reduces muscle soreness and that may enhance performance. MSM also helps you recover quicker from demanding physical exertion.

Appendix C

SELECTED REFERENCES

Books

Benjamin, Ben E. *Listen to Your Pain.* New York: Penguin Books, 1984.

Bonica, John J., ed. *The Management of Pain.* Philadelphia: Lea & Febiger, 1990.

Deichman, W. B., and H. W. Gerarde, eds. *Toxicology of Drugs & Chemicals,* Fourth Edition. New York: Academic Press, 1969.

Hannington-Kiff. *Pain Relief.* Philadelphia: J.B. Lippincott, 1974.

Heinerman, John. *The Healing Benefits of Garlic.* New Canaan, CT: Keats Publishing, Inc., 1994.

Huxtable, Ryan J. *Biochemistry of Sulfur.* New York: Plenum Press, 1986.

Jacob, S. W., E. E. Rosenbaum, and D. C. Wood. *Dimethyl Sulfoxide (Basic Concepts),* New York: Marcel Dekker, Inc., 1971.

Jacob, S. W., ed. *Biological Actions of Dimethyl Sulfoxide,* Volume 243. New York: New York Academy of Sciences, 1975.

Jacob, S. W., C. Francone, and W. Lossow. *Structure and Function in Man,* Fifth Edition, Philadelphia: W.B. Saunders and Co., 1982.

Jacob, S. W., R. J. Herschler, and H. Schmellenkamp. *The Use of DMSO in Medicine.* Munich: Springer Verlag, 1985.

Jacob, S. W., and J. G. Kappel. *DMSO.* Munich: Springer Verlag, 1988.

Jacob, S. W., and C. Francone. *Elements of Anatomy and Physiology.* Philadelphia: W.B. Saunders and Co., 1989.

Mitchell, Stephen C. *Biological Interactions of Sulfur Compounds.* Bristol, PA: Taylor & Francis, 1996.

Mussinan, Cynthia J., and Mary E. Keelan. *Sulfur Compounds in Foods.* Washington, DC: American Chemical Society, 1994.

Pfeiffer, Carl, *Mental and Elemental Nutrients.* New Canaan, CT: Keats Publishing, 1975.

Rapp, Doris. *Is This Your Child's World?* New York: Bantam Books, 1996.

Saltzman, Eric S., and William J. Cooper. *Biogenic Sulfur in the Environment.* Washington, DC: American Chemical Society, 1989.

Tarshis, Barry. *DMSO—The True Story of a Remarkable Pain-Killing Drug.* New York: Morrow, 1981.

Werbach, Melvyn R. *Nutritional Influences on Illness.* Tarzana, CA: Third Line Press, 1996.

Articles

American Medical Association. *Science News Updates,* "Pain reaches 'epidemic' proportions in the U.S.," July 17, 1997.

Associated Press. "A Breakthrough for Victims of Arthritis" *Los Angeles Times,* August 8, 1998, A4.

Astin, John A. "Education and health status predictors of alternative medicine usage," *Journal of the American Medical Association,* May 20, 1998, 279:1548–53.

Atcheson, Steven G., et al. "Concurrent medical disease in work-related carpal tunnel syndrome." *Archives of Internal Medicine,* 1998, 158:1506–12.

Bates, David W., et al. "Incidence of adverse drug events and potential adverse drug events." *Journal of the American Medical Association,* July 5, 1995, 274 (1):29.

Bauer, K., et al. "Pharmacodynamic effects of inhaled dry powder formulations of fenoterol and colforsin in asthma." *Clinical Pharmacology & Therapeutics,* 1993, 53 (1):76–83.

Bjarnason, I., et al. "Intestinal permeability and inflammation in rheumatoid arthritis: Effects of non-steroidal anti-inflammatory drugs." *Lancet,* 1984, 2:1171–74.

Brandsma, Maynard, et al. "Systemic lupus erythematosus." *Angiology,* 1970, 21 (3):172–78.

Castell, D. O., et al. "Gastroesophageal Reflux Disease: Current strategies for patient management." *Archives of Family Medicine,* 1996, 5:221–27.

Childs, Stacy. "Dimethyl sulfone (DMSO₂) in the treatment of interstitial cystitis." *Urologic Clinics of North America,* 1994, 21 (4).

Consumer Reports. "How is your doctor treating you?" February 1995, 81–88.

Deutsch, E. "Beeinflussung der blutgerinnung durch DMSO and kombinationen mit heparin." *DMSO Symposium, Vienna, 1966* (G. Laudahn and K. Gertich, eds.), Saladruck, Berlin, 1966, 144–49.

Deyo, Richard A. "Low-back pain." *Scientific American,* August 1998: 49–53.

DiPadova, S. "S-adenyl-methionine in the treatment of osteoarthritis: Review of clinical studies." *American Journal of Medicine,* 1987, 83, Supplement 5A:60–65.

Eaton, K. K., and A. Hunnisett. "Abnormalities in essential amino acids in patients with chronic fatigue syndrome." *Journal of Nutritional Medicine,* 1991, 2:369–78.

Eisenberg, D. M., et al. "Unconventional medicine in the United States." *New England Journal of Medicine,* January 28, 1993, 238:246–52.

Engle, M. F. "Indications and contraindications for the use of DMSO in clinical dermatology." *Annals of the New York Academy of Sciences,* 1967, 141:638–45.

———. "Dimethyl sulfoxide in the treatment of scleroderma." *Southern Medical Journal,* 1972, 65:71.

Evans, M. S., et al. "Dimethyl sulfoxide (DMSO) blocks conduction in peripheral nerve C fibers: a possible mechanism of analgesia." *Neuroscience Letters,* 1993, 150:145–48.

Fries, J. F., and S. R. Miller, et al. "Toward an epidemiology of gastropathy associated with nonsteroidal anti-inflammatory drug use." *Gastroenterology,* 1989, 96:647–55.

Fries, J. F., and C. A. Williams, et al. "Nonsteroidal anti-inflammatory drug-associated gastropathy: incidence and risk factor models." *American Journal of Medicine,* 1991, 91 (3):209–12.

Griffin, M. R. "Epidemiology of nonsteroidal anti-inflammatory drug-associated gastrointestinal injury." *American Journal of Medicine,* March 30, 1998, 104 (3A):23S-29S.

"Guidelines for the diagnosis and management of asthma." *Expert Panel Report No. 2,* 1997, National Institutes of Health (NIH Publication No. 97-4051).

Hoffman, Catherine, Dorothy, Rice, and Hai-Yen Sung. "Persons with chronic conditions." *Journal of the American Medical Association,* November 13, 1996, 276: 1473–79.

Holgate, Stephen T., and Anthony J. Frew. "Choosing therapy for childhood asthma." *New England Journal of Medicine,* 1997, 337 (23):1659–65.

Hucker, H. B., et al. "Studies on the absorption, excretion and metabolism of dimethyl sulfoxide (DMSO) in man." *Journal of Pharmacology and Experimental Therapeutics,* 1967, 155 (2):309–17.

Jacob, Stanley, and Robert Herschler. "Pharmacology of DMSO." *Cryobiology,* 1986, 23.

————. "Biological actions and medical applications of dimethyl sulfoxide." *Annals of the New York Academy of Sciences* (J. C. de la Torre, ed.), 1983, 411:xiii–xvii.

Johnson, Jeffrey A., and Lyle Bootman. "Drug-related morbidity and mortality: a cost-of-illness model." *Archives of Internal Medicine,* October 9, 1995, 155:1949–64.

Kamiya, S., et al. "Studies on improvement of eye drops." *Japan Journal of Clinical Ophthalmology,* 1966, 20: 143–52.

Kolata, Gina. "Study Raises Serious Doubts About Commonly Used Methods of Treating Back Pain." *The New York Times,* July 14, 1994.

Lawrence, R. M. "Methylsulfonylmethane (MSM): A double-blind study of its use in degenerative arthritis." *International Journal of Anti-Aging Medicine,* Summer 1998, 1 (1):50.

Layman, Don. "Growth inhibitory effects of dimethyl sulfoxide and dimethyl sulfone on vascular smooth muscle and endothelial cells in vitro." *In Vitro Cellular & Developmental Biology,* 1987, 23 (6):422–28.

Layman, Don, et al. "Suppression of atherosclerosis in cholesterolemic rabbits by dimethyl sulfoxide." *Annals of the New York Academy of Sciences,* 1983, 411:336–39.

Layman, Don, and Stanley Jacob. "The absorption, metabolism and excretion of dimethyl sulfoxide by rhesus monkeys." *Life Sciences,* 1985, 37:2431–37.

Lester, M. R. "Sulfite sensitivity: significance in human health." *Journal of the American College of Nutrition,* 1995, 14 (3):229–32.

Lovelock, J. E. "Atmospheric dimethyl sulphide and the natural sulphur cycle." *Nature,* 237, 1972, 452–53.

McCabe, Daniel, Eugene Woltering, et al. "Polar solvents in the chemoprevention of dimethylbenzanthracene-induced rat mammary cancer." *Archives of Surgery,* 1986, 121:1455–59.

Maibach, E. "On the influence of Japanese sulfur baths on degenerative arthritis." *Praxis,* 1966, 30:899–903.

Manga, P., D. Angus, et al. "The effectiveness and cost effectiveness of chiropractic management of low back pain." The Ontario Ministry of Health, Ottawa, Canada, August 1993.

Marcolongo R., et al. "Double-blind multicenter study of the activity of S-adenylmethionine in hip osteoarthritis." *Current Therapeutic Research,* 1985, 37: 82–94.

Martin, W., "Natuerliches vorkommen vom dimethylsulfoxide and dimethylsulfon im menschlichen organismus." *International DMSO Workshop Hannover,* September 19, 1987 (S. W. Jacob and J. E. Kappel, eds.), W. Zuckschwerdt Publishing, Munich/San Francisco, 1988:71–77.

Metcalf, John, "MSM—A dietary derivative of DMSO," *Equine Veterinary Data,* 3 (5), 1983:148, 174–75.

Milne, P. J., et al. "Rate of reaction of methanesulfonic acid, dimethyl sulfoxide, and dimethyl sulfone with hydroxyl radical in aqueous solution." *Biogenic Sulfur in the Environment* (Eric S. Saltzman, William J. Cooper, eds.), American Chemical Society, Washington, DC, 1989, 518–28.

Monmaney, Terrance, and Shari Roan. "Alternative medicine—the $18 billion experiment." *Los Angeles Times,* August 30, 1998, p. 1.

Moore, R. D., and J. I. Morton. "Diminished inflammatory joint disease in MRL/1pr mice ingesting dimethyl sulfoxide (DMSO) or methyl-sulfonylmethane (MSM)." Federation of American Societies for Experimental Biology, 69th annual meeting, April 1985, p. 692.

Moore, Thomas J., et al. "U.S. drug safety monitoring must be expanded." *Journal of the American Medical Association,* 1998, 279:1571–73.

Morton, Jane I., R. D. Moore, and S. W. Jacob. "DMSO or MSM in the drinking water of mice protect against the development of hemolytic anemia and immune complex renal disease." Unpublished study.

Morton, Jane I., and R. D. Moore. "Lupus nephritis and deaths are diminished in B/W mice drinking 3% water solutions of dimethyl sulfoxide (DMSO) and dimethyl sulfone ($DMSO_2$)." *Journal of Leukocyte Biology,* 1986, 40 (3):322.

Morton, Jane I., and Benjamin V. Siegel. "Effects of oral dimethyl sulfoxide and dimethyl sulfone on murine autoimmune lymphoproliferative disease." *Proceedings of the Society for Experimental Biology and Medicine,* 1986, 183:227–30.

Moss, Jeffrey. "A perspective on sulfur—Is it the most ignored, misunderstood essential trace element." *The Moss Nutrition Report,* August 1997, Hadley, MA.

Mudd, S. H. "Sixteen inherited human diseases are now recognized, affecting most of the major steps in sulphur metabolism." *Sulphur in Biology,* CIBA Foundation Symposium 72, Excerpta Medica, 1980, 239.

"New guidelines on managing chronic pain in older persons." Medical News and Perspectives, *Journal of the American Medical Association,* July 22/29, 1998.

O'Dwyer, Patrick, et al. "Use of polar solvents in chemoprevention of 1,2-dimethylhydrazine-induced colon cancer." *Cancer,* 1988, 62: 944–48.

Osterberg, E. E., et al. "Absorption of sulfur compounds during treatment by sulfur baths." *Archives Dermatol Syphilol,* 1929, 20:156–66.

Pearson, Thomas W. "Natural occurring levels of dimethyl sulfoxide in selected fruits, vegetables, grains and beverages." *Journal of Agricultural and Food Chemistry,* 1981, 29:1089.

Perez-Marrero, R., et al. "A controlled study of dimethyl sulfoxide in interstitial cystitis." *Journal of Urology,* 1988, 140:36–39.

Pfiffner, J. J., and H. B. North. "Dimethyl sulfone: A constituent of the adrenal gland." *Journal of Biological Chemistry,* 1940, 131:731.

Potterton, D. "The politics of asthma: Out of control." *Nursing Times,* 1992, 88 (2): 26–31.

Pottz, G. E., et al. "Die verwendung von DMSO zur schellfarbung von mykobakterien and anderen mikroorganismen in abstrichen and gewebeschnitten." *DMSO Symposium, Vienna, 1966* (G. Laudahand, K. Gertich, eds.), Saladruck, Berlin, 1966, 40–43.

Richmond, V. L. "Incorporation of methylsulfonylmethane sulfur into guinea pig serum proteins." *Life Sciences,* 1986, 39:263–68.

Rizzo, R. "Calcium sulfur and zinc distribution in normal and arthritic articular equine cartilage: A Syncrotron radiation induced X-ray emission study." *Journal of Experimental Zoology,* Sept. 1995, 237 (1):82–86.

Ruzicka, L., et al. "Isolation of dimethyl sulfone from cow's blood." *Helvetica Chimica Acta.,* 1940, 23:559–61.

Scherbel, A. L., L. J. McCormack, and J. K. Layle. "Further observations on the effect of dimethyl sulfoxide in patients with generalized scleroderma (progressive systemic sclerosis)." *Annals of the New York Academy of Sciences,* 1967, 141:613–29.

Schroeder, Henry. "Losses of vitamins and trace minerals resulting from processing and preservation of foods." *American Journal of Clinical Nutrition,* 1971, 24:562–73.

Scott, D. L., Coulton, B. L., et al. "Long-term outcome of treating rheumatoid arthritis: Results after 20 years." *Lancet,* 1989: 1108–11.

Senturia, Ben. "Results of treatment of chronic arthritis and rheumatoid conditions with colloidal sulfur." *Journal of Bone and Joint Surgery,* 1934, 16:119–25.

Shealy, C. N. "The physiological substrate of pain." *Headache,* 1966, 6:101–8.

Shield, M. J. "Anti-inflammatory drugs and their effects on cartilage synthesis and renal function." *European Journal of Rheumatoid Inflammation,* 1993, 13:7–16.

Smith, Robert. "Diagnosing headache." *Hospital Medicine,* 1997, 33 (7):26–42.

Steely, Jeffrey S. "Chemiluminescence detection of sulfur compounds in cooked milk," in *Sulphur Compounds in Foods.* Mussinan & Keelan, eds. American Chemical Society, Washington, DC, 1994, 8.

Sullivan, M. S., and W. C. Hess. "Cystine content in fingernails in arthritics." *Journal of Bone Joint Surgery,* 1935, 16:185–88.

U.S. Agency for Health Care Policy and Research. "Acute Low Back Problems in Adults." *Clinical Practice Guideline No. 14,* 1994.

Volpi, Elena, et al. "Exogenous amino acids stimulate net muscle protein synthesis in the elderly." *Journal of Clinical Investigation,* 1998, 101 (9):2000–2007.

Weissman, G., et al. "Effect of DMSO on the stabilization of lysosomes by cortisone and chloroquine in vitro." *Annals of the New York Academy of Science,* 1967, 141:326–32.

Williams, K.I.H. "Dimethyl sulfone: Isolation from cows' milk." *Proceedings of the Society for Experimental Biology & Medicine,* 1966, 122:865.

Williams, K.I.H., et al. "Dimethyl sulfone: Isolation from human urine." *Archives of Biochemistry and Biophysics,* 1966, 113:251–52.

Woldenberg, S. C. "The treatment of chronic arthritis & rheumatoid conditions with colloidal sulfur." *Journal of the Southern Medical Association,* 1935, 28:875–81.

Young, Vernon R., and Antoine E. El-Khoury, "The notion of the nutritional essentiality of amino acids, revisited, with a note on the indispensable amino acid requirements in adults," in *Amino Acid Metabolism and Therapy in Health and Nutritional Disease* (Luc Cynober, ed.), CRC Press, Boca Raton, 1995, 213–14.

Zucker, Martin. "It's in your hands: Treating repetitive strain injuries with herbs, supplements and body therapies." *Vegetarian Times,* May 1998:22.

———. "Homocysteine Update," *Let's Live Magazine,* April 1998:44–48.

Index